No
WHITE
Diet !

"A Lifestyle for Fast and Healthy Weight Loss "

Paul Array

D1400983

ISBN: 1-4196-6633-9
ISBN- 13: 978-141966633-9
Library of Congress Control Number: 2007902664
Publisher: Booksurge, LLC
North Charleston, South Carolina

Disclaimer

Before starting any diet, lifestyle program, serious change in eating habits or exercise program, individuals should consult with their physician or primary health provider. All information in this book and/ or accompanying materials is of a general nature and is furnished for educational purposes only. No information contained in this book or in any accompanying materials is to be taken as medical or other health advice pertaining to any individual's specific health or medical condition. The information is not a diagnosis, treatment plan, or recommendation for a particular course of action regarding your health and is not intended to provide specific medical advice.

The Creators, advisors, consultants, editors, wholesalers, distributors and retailers are not liable or responsible, in whole or in part, to any person or entity for any injury, damage, or loss of any sort caused or alleged to be caused directly or indirectly by the use, practice, teaching, or other dissemination of any of the techniques, recommendations, information or ideas presented in this book or accompanying materials.

It remains your sole responsibility to evaluate the accuracy, completeness, and usefulness of the information provided by the " No White Diet ."

Notice

This book is intended as a reference volume only, not as a medical manual. It is not intended as a substitute for any treatment that may have been prescribed by your doctor. If you suspect that you have a medical problem, we urge you to seek competent medical help. This book is sold with the understanding that the authors and publishers are not engaging in direct person-to-person advice.
Mention of specific companies, organizations, or authorities in this book does not imply endorsement by the publisher or author, nor does mention of specific companies, organizations, or authorities imply that they endorse this book.

Acknowledgments

Way up there on the top of the list to acknowledge and thank is my wife Mardy. She has stuck with me through all my diets and all my fads. She has cooked many meals from a great number of cookbooks trying to help me lose weight. Mardy has always encouraged me to keep my heart healthy by teaching me, how to exercise properly, eat correctly and take my vitamins. She has always encouraged me.
Thank you Mardy.

There should be words greater then ' Thanks ' for the people that are so gracious to give a most precious commodity, their time, to help me with this book. Walter A. Morin Phd., professor in Emeritus. Noreen Sofranac RD LD Nutritionist. Karen Kelly MA in development and clinical Psychology specializing in eating disorders. Oh…. how lucky I am to have found people like this.
Thank you, Thank you, Thank you.

Preface

This preface will probably be different than most you have read; then again this book is probably different than *any* you have read. There must be 100,000 diet books on the market, why should this one stand out from any of the others? The food hasn't changed since the last book was put on the market, has it? Why is this book different than the rest? Because I am a simple guy without fancy credentials who has finally learned the art of staying healthy. I can spare you the headaches of learning the hard way, and save you lots of dollars and time in your search for the right plan.

Besides, I finally accepted the fact that eating must be a pleasurable experience..... every day. The way I eat needs to be worked into my lifestyle and has to include all the great flavors. (*I would much rather collect cookbooks than diet books any day*)

Let me tell you off the record...... how much I am bothered by thin doctors and pretty personal trainers trying to tell fat guys like me how I should eat. In my opinion thin people do not have the same urges as us fat people. Do they know about desires to eat at 4 in the afternoon or the difficulties staying motivated to exercise? I don't think so.

Over the years of dieting I have found that the problem is deeper than just what food to eat. Walk around the grocery store and look at the people. Check out their carts when they're unloading them at the register. People just do not know what to buy. I think they're confused while shopping and so they just pick what they have eaten for years, (*i.e. comfort food*) I hardly see anyone looking at the labels before they place the packages of food in their cart. Why? Because they're confused. After all, the labels are almost impossible to read unless you're a nutritionist.

I am going to show you how to shop, how to read those labels and then I'm going to tell you how to make good food choices. After all, whenever I was confused I would fall back on comfort food like everyone else.

Secondly, I am going to teach you in plain english how the digestive system works and what it takes to keep the weight from creeping back. All of us have lost weight just to put it back on again in a relatively short amount of time. Getting a handle on those hunger cravings is another secret we will tackle.

Do you need a diet plan, portion controls, three exact meals a day, a calorie counter, food supplements, a person watching you weigh yourself each week? NO. You're more intelligent that that. By the way, diet plans don't work either because most people can't possibly stay on them long enough to matter. Sure, they will work for the short run but will you stick with them? I couldn't.

Buying pre packaged food from a diet company can make dieting a breeze but it costs you a lot of money. Then on top of selling you the food, they charge you a subscription fee. (*Hello!!*) Don't get wrapped around that finger.

What is the answer? The answer is in the pages that follow. We are going to change our lifestyle. We are going to know what to buy, how to buy it and we are, most of all, going to eat delicious food without portion controls, that will fill us up but still allow us to lose weight faster than most diets.

You know what else? You're going to be happy while you're eating. You're even going to be happy shopping for the food because you will be an educated consumer.

You're NOT going to believe all those commercials trying to sell you the magic pill. You're not going to believe the diet commercials telling you that you can lose 20 pounds in 20 days. (*who are they kidding ?*) You are certainly not going to believe that if you buy that exercise machine and only use it 5 minutes a day in 6 weeks you will have the greatest body on earth.

Be realistic. We are going to change our ways or we are not going to sustain the weight loss.

That said .... Let's get on with it !

CONTENTS

No
WHITE
Diet !

Part One

LET'S BE HONEST

Am I a Doctor ? No
Am I a Nutrition expert ? No
Am I a Health Care Professional ? No
Do I know how to lose weight ? **Yes**
Can I help you lose weight and keep the weight off ? **Yes**
Can I guarantee that you will keep the weight off, be slim and trim with great abs and a perfect body ? No
Do you need to exercise to lose weight with this diet ? No, but it helps.
Will you be healthy ? **Yes**
Will you be happy with yourself? **Yes**

I'm just a fat guy that has a hard time losing weight. I will say that reading some of the diet books out there and listening to thin guys on the tube telling me how to lose weight really irks me. In my opinion, a thin person never had the urges a fat person has and never will. I should make it one of my rules, ' Beware of the thin people telling you how to lose weight'.

If you want to hear the truth, read on. If you're one of those people that likes to be told fairy tales, put this book back on the shelf. You don't need me, you need a head doctor before you start a weight loss program.

How about we combine three of the right things to do. Eat right, do a little activity and lose some weight? And by the way..... let's do this without suffering. Toss the heavy guilt aside and start living. Read this book only if you're in a good mood. Make this fun.

I have done every diet imaginable. The low calorie, low sugar, low carb, popcorn, hawaiian, Mediterranean, zone, pasta, greek, surfers, Atkins, Sugar Busters, South Beach, caribbean, dessert, cranberry, lemonade, celery, Heart Association, etc., etc. I even took xenical (to get rid of fat in food) prescribed by my doctor/ cardiologist. I have been doing cardiovascular exercising 5 days a week for 5 years. I always wear a heart rate monitor while exercising to stay in the Zone. *(more on that later)*. Then I would do my weight exercises. *(three days a week)*. Did the diets work ? NO ....Did the exercise help ? It kept my heart healthy but I ate too much and mostly the wrong things to lose weight.

1

Why didn't any of this work? Because I did not stick with any of them. Of course some of them, like the pineapple or popcorn diet for example, were really getting boring. I mean....how many different ways can you fix pineapple? Bottom line!.. Forget about diets. I should say, forget about the word diet. Diets do not work. What works is a life style change. If you are willing to change your eating habits, (*I did not say suffer*), then let me turn you on to some great eating, delicious food and weight loss you will be happy with. Yes....... Happy! If you're happy then I'm happy,

If you are not willing to change your eating habits then again I advise you to put this book back on the shelf.(*That's the second time I told you to do that, maybe you should listen?) (Then you can tell everyone that the* " No White Diet " *book doesn't work :>)*

There is no sense putting good money after bad money. I am sure you have bought all the other books on the market. I certainly have. Why buy this one if you don't really want to do it.

Ahhhhhhhhh...................your still here ! Good

In a nutshell I promise you this:
 " You will learn to eat guilt free " (*won't that make us happy?)*

" Exercise will not be a big focus here, (*unless of course you want it to. :>)* although it's important for well being ",

" The food I suggest will taste great. "

" Can I still eat at fast food establishments? " Of course!

" No preaching about portion controls", (*well....... maybe that's a lie but it's just a little white lie)*

" You will find those cravings to eat disappearing. "

" You will be a " happy puppy' after you start this diet. "

Did I say Diet........... DIET!!....... yes , I said it. The reason I use the word is because I can't find a better one. Besides that, Diet books sell well and I want to sell this one. So.....................until one of you write to me with a better word I will use it throughout this book although I think Life Style Change is what this is all about. The problem with using Life Style Change for the title of the book is that you would never buy the book.

Just imagine if I named it 'Don't Diet, Life Style Change it'. Would you buy it? Of course not. I wouldn't either.

I have some rules that you are going to need to learn. Only 4 of them. They're simple and they will be everything you need to know to lose weight.

The one thing I do not want to do is get complicated. One of my pet peeves is a Doctor, especially a thin Doctor, writing a diet book. They seem to be writing for other Doctors'. How can the rest of us average people understand all their gibberish? They talk funny. Did you ever try to understand a doctor? I go in to get an examination and sometimes I have to ask him twice what he's talking about. This book is written for the average person. You do not need to know all the technical jargon they try to tell you. I will tell you everything you need to know about losing weight. I will tell it in a simple, easy to understand manner using words we all know. (another pet peeve, Big Words)

By the way, I started off with a blood cholesterol level of over 300 and triglycerides close to 300. *(should be under 200)* My good cholesterol was much worse then my bad. My blood pressure was high and I felt like I was being flushed down a toilet. I now have a cholesterol count of under 110 with triglycerides also under 110, my good cholesterol is much higher then my bad. My blood pressure is 110 over 78 and the toilet tank is filling. I took a stress test at my cardiologists office *(My wife was harping on me to do it, 'age' she said)* and he said, " If you die it won't be because of your heart."

Does my diet work, you tell me !

Why is the Book called "No White Diet"

I started out with the name ' Key West Lifestyle Diet', probably because I live in Key West and the people that come here are always active and seem to have the right lifestyle. *(although they drink too much)* I thought it was a good name but friends told me that is was not catchy enough. *(what do they know)*

I then came up with the name 'Tell the Truth Diet'. I wanted to tell everyone the real truth about dieting so it seemed appropriate. After thinking about it for weeks upon weeks I decided that it was pretty dumb. Why should you think I was telling you the truth when nobody else was. Actually a lot of diet books are telling you the truth.

One day I was sitting in a little Cafe (Jerry's Cafe) on Commercial Blvd. in Fort Lauderdale with some friends of mine, Larry and Donna Dearman. The discussion came around to me. "What have you been doing lately, Paul", " Just finishing my diet, lifestyle book" I said.

I was perplexed at the time as to what I should name the book, various names swimming in my head. My friends listened regarding the content and reasons for writing the book. After much discussion during lunch we left to go in our own directions. About 10 minutes later I received a phone call on my cell phone from Donna with the name 'Don't Die-it, Live it'.

After soul searching the name for a few days I decided to use it. Why? It typifies exactly what I am trying to tell each and every one of you. Obesity is a disease that has to be stopped. We need to eat better and get to a weight level where we are within the guidelines for a healthy body.

I kept the name for quite some time until I realized that it just wouldn't sell. Before going to the publisher I changed it to 'No White Diet'. Why?........... read on. *(bet you'll find out why)*

Get Excited !

During the research for the book I met (by phone) a psychologist and nutritionist from New York. After a long discussion I found out why he thinks people buy Diet books. The reasoning surprised me.

He believes from all the people interviewed and spoken to during his tour as a public speaker, that most people who are overweight are not happy. That people are looking for a book that will make them happy while they are trying to lose weight.

I want to make you happy. I do not want it to be drudgery for you to lose weight and get in better shape. We need to make this fun, we need to get excited, so let's do that. Look at this book as a fun book. Attitude is everything. If you decide you're going to have fun, then you will. We're going to learn about food, the digestive system, how to shop and we're going to lose weight. Remember, I am right along side you, the fat guy, always trying to lose weight.

You are going to be happy because you are shedding the pounds. You're going to feel good about yourself. Your clothes are going to start feeling big. Won't this be great ? Darn right it will. Get EXITED !

Emotion plays a huge part in the weight loss equation. If you're sad, down in the dumps, depressed, or going thru a rough period in your life you won't lose weight. You're going to eat more. This is not the time to try a life style change. Get your emotions in check. Look at this life style change as a positive emotion.

If you feel that you have a problem and I might be able to help you with it, e-mail me and let me answer your question. Just go to the website at www.nowhitediet.com and click on contact us. If you need a structured diet plan or just want more recipes, please visit our web site.

A Few Statistics

Let's look at some statistics about how much weight the American people have gained over the past 20 years.

The column on the right represents the number of States in which the people were more then 30 pounds overweight. Each color represents the percentage of people overweight in each state.

▨ 10% of People ■ 15% of People ■ 20% of People
▨ 25% of People ■ 30% of People ░ 35% of People

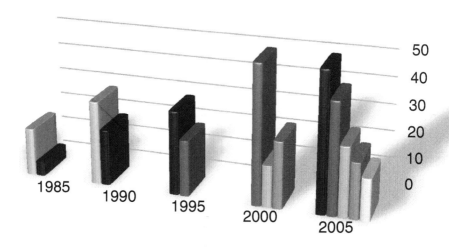

Example: in 1985 10% of the people were overweight in 10 states and 15% of the people were overweight in 5 states. Look at the increase in 2005 !

In 2005 15% of the people were overweight in 48 of the states. 20% of the people were overweight in 35 states. 25% of the people were over-weight in 20 states and 35% of the people were overweight in 10 states.

This is a dramatic increase in just 20 years. What's going to happen in the next 10 years? Are 50% of our people going to be more then 30 pounds overweight in all the states ? This is a frightening number that we have to combat now.

Looking at these statistics on a different type of graph; the following table, starting in 1985, shows how quickly the the percentage of population in the United States has increased in weight. The column on the right is the number of states.

The upper line indicates that 10% of the people were more then 30 pounds overweight in 10 states in 1985. In 2005 10% of the people in all 50 states are overweight.
The lower line reveals the fact that 35% of the people were more then 30 pounds overweight in only 3 states in 1990 but in 2005 35% of the people were more then 30 pounds overweight in over 15 states. Project that into the future and in 10 years 35% of the people will be overweight in all **50** States.

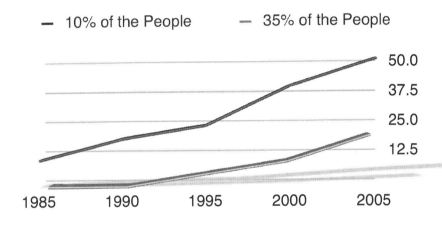

— 10% of the People   — 35% of the People

50.0
37.5
25.0
12.5

1985   1990   1995   2000   2005

This is really an unexceptable figure. It needs to change. Hopefully, you are not going to be part of these statistics anymore. Are you?

In all seriousness it seems that the problem has compounded itself since the influx of fast food. Not only the fast food from restaurants like Mc Donald's, Burger King, KFC or Pizza Hut but the fast food we all eat every day. We don't just eat it for lunch but also for breakfast and dinner. Our lifestyles are changing, more and more family's have both the parents working. When they get home from a long hard day, cooking is about the last thing anyone want's to do. Consequently, a quick meal is usually the preferred choice.

I understand that problem and have tried to introduce quick dinners that are still good for you. Take a look at the recipes under part two.

For breakfast there are ways to eat healthy even if you just have a slice of whole grain toast and a glass of V8 or some other low calorie, low sugar vegetable juice. I have included recipes for breakfast that are fast and nutritious.

Please, let's change this statistic.

Is there a Magic Pill ?

No, and don't let anyone tell you there is. Forget the written advertisements and infomercials. The only way to lose weight is to either keep your mouth closed or change your eating habits. If you do the research you will find that the diets that work for the long run are the ones which change your eating habits.

Example: Jenny Craig or Weight Watchers. They proportion the food and give you low calorie, low fat food. Are they right ? Of course they are but most of us cannot or won't do it. I emphasis the Won't. It's too restrictive and quite expensive. Trying to feed a family of 4 or 6 on one of those diets would bankrupt a lot of people. I truly believe that we can all lose weight with a minimum amount of expense.

Is there a pill that can help ? YES It's called Xenical (orlistat) and it is a prescription medicine that blocks the absorption of about ¼ of any fat consumed. You take it while eating. There are warnings with this medicine and you need to discuss the implications with your doctor before taking it. I do know it has a warning for pregnant woman and woman that are breast feeding. Does it work ? Yes it does, I took it for a couple of years with minimal side effects. Since it helps to stop the absorption of fat some people think it's a pill you can take and then eat fatty food. NO, NO, NO. Then you are defeating the purpose of taking the pill. If your going to take it, you need to also eat non fatty food.

Now let me explain the bad part about taking the pill. Two things. First, is it can cause diarrhea and / or very soft stool. Secondly, there is yellow liquid associated with the soft stool that is really all the fat that would have gone into your body. The only way to disburse the yellow liquid is to NOT eat food with a lot of fat in it and one trick is to take fiber pills with the Xenical. I took Fiber Choice. Available in any Pharmacy. You take one Xenical and 2 fiber pills. Go to Xenical.com and read about it.

Oh Yea, forgot one thing. Lot's of gas with this pill. LOT'S of gas.

On February 7, 2007 The government approved over-the-counter sales of the fat-blocking diet pill Orlistat, allowing direct sales for the first time of a version of the diet drug Xenical that had been available only by prescription. Currently available as Xenical, the capsules will be sold in a lower, nonprescription dose under the name "Alli "

Do you need this Orlistat ? If you follow what I am about to tell you in this book, No. You will shed pounds with out any artificial or medical stimulation.

By the way, when they come out with a true magic pill I will be the first to try it and then I will pass the information on to you.

But first.......... I get to use it. Fair Deal ?

The Great Secret to all Diets

First, I'm going to explain to you the greatest secret in all diets. (*I'm climbing on my soap box now*). The one thing that no one wants to tell you. It doesn't matter what diet you are on, what they tell you, or how you go about it. There is only one thing you have to do to lose weight. You could write a new diet book and make a lot of money with this amazing secret. Ready ?........

Rule #1: Keep your mouth closed !

Yep, that's it. The one way to absolutely lose weight on any diet you are on. If you stop eating, or I should say, slow down your eating you will lose weight.

Can we do that ? Obviously Not. If you could do it then you would not be reading this book. I am here to help you with keeping your mouth closed, or at least sometimes. To teach you how to eat. How to stay full and yet lose weight. Too good to be true ? Not really..............stay with me.

If you listen, you will not only lose weight but you will keep it off and that is the important part of my way of eating. The pounds do not come back on again. I can't count how many times I have lost weight, just to put it back on again.

Now.............let us get started.

Let's look at the Europeans

I had a chance to spend summers in Europe working on a Sailboat. I noticed that especially in France the people were much slimmer than the Americans I knew. Even in Italy, where pasta is the mainstay, people were still not as fat as I was.

What…….. is going on here ?

The reason for this is simple. There life style is different. They are taught at a very young age how to eat. Do they eat fast food ? No. Do they eat food with Fat ? Yes. Do they eat carbs ? Yes. Then why aren't they fat ? Because they eat the right kind of fat and their portion size is smaller. After spending 12 summers in the Mediterranean I got the idea. (*takes me a while to catch on, doesn't it?*) Every summer that I was in the Med I would lose weight. Would I eat carbs like fresh bread and pasta ? Yes. Would I eat meat like steak, pork and lamb? Yes. Would I eat potatoes? very seldom. Even fried potatoes? Yes (*fried, just once in a great while*) Still, I lost weight.

Reliable studies have confirmed that low rates of coronary artery disease occur in Mediterranean countries where the population consumes a large percentage of their calories in monounsaturated fats, primarily in the form of Olive oil. Also, beneficial effects come from walnuts and almonds. Does this mean eat all the almonds or walnuts you like ? NO, but a few a day are good for you. A mediterranean- type diet should be high in vegetables, fresh fruit, whole grains and olive oil.

The secret……. lean meats, very small amounts of fried food (fried in the right oil) heavy hearty bread (small portion) made with whole grains and a glass or 2 of wine each night. (*I like that part*)

I find, lately, since the US has invaded the Europeans with fast food restaurants like Mc Donald's, Burger King , Kentucky Fried Chicken and Pizza Hut that they are starting to raise their body fat. Is it because of the restaurants ? I can answer that by saying "it is because they are starting to eat wrong, just like us". You can do it in any restaurant if your not careful. It is not the fault of the fast food chains.
It is OUR fault for eating wrong. Don't blame the restaurant, Blame yourself for breaking rule Number 1.

Is Alcohol always bad for you?

We have all heard how fattening alcohol is. Now, I am going to tell you that this is only partially true. Compared to other carbohydrates, alcohol is far less fattening. *(except Beer, Beer is reeeeeeeeeally fattening)* Look at it this way. When you eat that sandwich and you have two slices of bread, get rid of one slice and have a glass of red wine. (4 ounces) Fewer calories then the slice of bread and better for you. The body uses alcohol as instant energy and as long as you drink it with food (specifically proteins) you won't receive what some say is the negative effect. *(some say that alcohol will not allow the body to burn fat from reserves)*

It should be said that some forms of alcohol are much worse then others. Beer is one of them. I would suggest you trash the beer and start drinking wine. *(Not so bad is it?)* Wine is perhaps the most acceptable form of alcohol. It has been shown that the death rate from heart attacks is lowest in countries where wine is habitually consumed, such as Italy, France and Spain.

Here's the bottom line, if your going to drink , then drink red wine and if your going to drink red wine , drink it after you eat protein. *(like a piece of meat or cheese)*

Don't start telling people that you read this diet book and the guy said I could drink all the red wine I wanted and lose weight.   :>)

One thing I know for sure. Alcohol consumption does not help you with weight loss. I will also say I have seen significant quantities of weight loss while consuming alcohol like that contained in Red Wine. Personally I believe that Red Wine helps in weight loss. After looking at the French people (one of the highest consumers of red wine) and speaking with them at length I suggest that a small amount of Red Wine per day is good for you.

How do I know so much about Diets

To be honest with you, I don't. Since I am not a skinny guy I said to myself I was going to find out. I am a researcher. I pride myself in turning over every rock if I have to learn something. I also have friends that are doctors, nutritionists and experts in eating disorders.

After 27 years of trying to lose weight, I can tell you I have turned over all the rocks in the Diet world. When I decided to write this book it took an immense amount of time to be sure of my thoughts.

Besides.................. I then had to lose weight and keep it off just to prove to myself that I was right. Am I now a thin guy. NO. But I am not as fat as I was and I'm very healthy. *(I am also in the Social Security bracket so you know my approximate age)*

Healthy is important.

A little about Diets in General

It is not my intent to try and tell you 'all the other diets on the market' don't work. After all, they all work if you can stick with them and refuse to return to your old ways. Probably the fastest way to lose weight is to have a band surgically put around your stomach or even having your stomach stapled. This generally works for truly morbid obese people who have an extreme amount of weight to lose. It works because you cant eat. Back to rule #1 Keep your mouth closed. This type of operation supports my first rule without any help from your brain.

Let's look at some of the other diets and see why they will not work for us. (*me especially*)

Perhaps the most famous, back in the 80's and 90's was the American Heart Association's recommended way of eating properly. Remember the pyramid? Low fat and high carbohydrates. There are many authors on the low fat, high carbohydrate type of eating. I won't bore you with all of their writings. I could not make it work and I thought after a couple of years it might be because of the carbs. (*read on and you will see why*)

Low fat diets that say you have to practically become a vegetarian to lose weight are just wrong. After all, what is wrong with meat? And how about Eggs? Something wrong with them also? I never believed that meat and eggs were the wrong thing to eat. I also need to have some dessert. After all, 'I deserve it and I am going to have it'. (*So…. There !*)

The next diet I tried and probably still the most famous is the Atkins Diet. Does it work ? Yes. My problem was I just couldn't keep eating the meats without the buns and no vegetables. No pasta either. (*my Mother would not like that. She was born in Italy*) My brain was so ingrained to not eating large quantities of fat that I just could not do it ! I finally quit . Great for the short run but in my opinion it is just not something I can stick with for the long haul. I would lose weight then gain it back.

The fad diets (*as I call them*) like the popcorn diet, pineapple diet, pasta diet are just what the sign says, Fads. I could not stand eating 14 different popcorns for 2 weeks or 37 ways to eat pineapple for that matter. Now……Pasta! I can eat some pasta, let me tell you. Problem was I couldn't lose weight with it. (*what a shame*)

The Zone diet. A doctor friend of mine turned me on to it. Does it work? Absolutely. What happened? it was just too complicated for me to remember. All those zones and portioning out all the food and counting, counting, measuring. Yuk !

The old count the calories Diet. Yep ! I did that for a while, use to carry a calorie book in my back pocket. Then came another book I had to carry because the first book didn't have all the foods in it. I would go into a restaurant and start looking at the menu and counting the calories on a napkin. It became silly. I was not going to start carrying an adding machine to lose weight.

How about the Sugar Busters Diet? Right on! Will it work? Yes. Trying to read the book is almost impossible unless you're a doctor. Of course it's written by a doctor. (*In fact, four of them. Can you imagine getting four doctors to agree on anything? Good for them. I can't get one person to agree, let alone four.*) I am a layman, not a doctor and books should be written for the average person. I had a hard time grasping what the guy was saying. If you can't understand the written word, you just cannot put it into practice.

Then came the South Beach Diet. What do I think ? *Pretty darn good diet. It works. I like it.* I like mine better. Why? because I am not going to ask you to carry a list of food numbers (glycemic index) around with you so you can eat the right items. I am also not going to try and sell you a diet plan. Compare the two and you might pick mine also. *(then again you might pick theirs. If you do.... good luck)*

The object here is to be healthy and lose weight. If someone else's diet floats your boat, then do it. I congratulate you for your weight loss and I would appreciate you contacting me and telling me so.

It's Important to know about Carbohydrates, Protein, Fat and Fiber.

Everything we eat is either a carbohydrate, protein, fat or fiber. Carbohydrates are broken down to simple sugar. (Actually about 80 percent glucose and 20% galactose or fructose depending on whether we had dairy products or fruit.) Proteins are broken down to amino acids. Fats are broken down to fatty acids (FA. Their simplest form triglycerides contain 3 FA's. Fiber is not broken down. The first three are absorbed into our body through the digestive tract. Fiber is not absorbed. Let's learn about the first three. (*Don't get bored, this is important)*

Carbohydrates come from both plants and animals. Most are from sugars and starches. Since the carbohydrates are converted into mostly glucose then lets look at carbohydrates as the fuel that feeds the body. When you're eating, the glucose is either used immediately or stored as fat to be used later. (*See why I told you to stay away from sugar?)*
When the level of glucose in your blood starts to drop, the body takes some of that stored glucose (actually called glycogen when stored) and raises the blood sugar level. If it rises too high then your body releases insulin to control it. (*more later on insulin)*

Proteins come from meats, nuts, dairy products and even some vegetables. Proteins broken down by enzymes secreted by the pancreas are reduced to amino acids. They can then be absorbed from the intestine. Amino Acids can be converted by the liver into Glucose. Mmmmmmmm......here's that word sugar again. Bottom line is that Glucose is what runs our bodies.

Fats come from both animals and vegetables. Yes, vegetables. (*Avocado has quite a bit of Fat (fairly good fat) so don't binge on the Guacamole*) Fats are broken down by pancreatic enzymes into fatty acids. But even broken down they have a hard time being absorbed. Our body, being as smart as it is provides a way for the fats to be absorbed. It's called bile, produced by the liver and stored in the gallbladder. It is used to break down large fat molecules into small fat molecules so they can be better absorbed. Don't get me wrong, fats are important for the body to use in the manufacture of cells. Another reason for fat is to provide a layer of insulation underneath the skin. Of course this layer should be thin. (*Obviously my layer is way too big.)*

Fibers: Remember this, when you eat any of the above you must eat fiber with it so the carbohydrates, proteins and fats are not absorbed quickly into the blood. One of our objects is to limit the carbohydrates, proteins and fats and eat more fiber.

The next chapter will tell you more.

It's more important to know about Insulin

I have broached the subject of Insulin a few times. Now it is time to get a little technical with you. Why? because you need to understand how the body digests food so you can actually see what to eat and what not to eat and how everything you eat gets distributed. (*Whew !*)

Here we go ! Insulin prevents the sugar level (glucose) from rising to high in the blood. Glucagon *(I know, I know, another one of those words)* is also secreted by the pancreas and prevents the blood sugar from falling to low. Glucagon really comes into effect if you were going to try to fast or starve yourself. During the first day you try to starve the liver can sustain you by taking Glucagon and converting the glycogen (stored glucose) into glucose. After you use up what's stored in the liver the Glucagon starts converting muscle protein into blood sugar. Not a good thing to happen and that is why you shouldn't try to starve yourself. (*No chance, Huh ?) (I tried that type of diet too, didn't work.*)

Most overweight people are over-producing insulin which overtime leads to an insulin fatigue of sorts and has been labeled insulin resistance. High insulin levels promotes the storage of sugar in the liver and in the muscles. Insulin also prevents the breakdown of triglycerides or fat. It becomes very hard for the person with high insulin levels to lose weight. With insulin resistance your fat cells, liver cells and muscle cells have become insensitive to normal levels of insulin. Usually a small amount of insulin will lower blood sugar. With insulin resistance this does not occur. Insulin activates an enzyme that removes fats (tryglycerides) from the blood and deposits them in fat cells. It also stimulates another enzyme that breaks down stored fats. Without these two activities you have an increase in stored fat. (*There is some evidence that maintaining a high Insulin level by having a high intake of carbs can "burn" out the pancreatic cells that make Insulin.*) Without getting more complicated you can see that when insulin is not playing it's part in the digestive system we gain or retain weight.

Ok, how do we correct this problem and reduce insulin resistance. Simple, we have to eat less of the insulin stimulating carbohydrates.

What are the most insulin Stimulating Carbohydrates? The big Kahuna is Beer. The fastest blood sugar riser is Maltose (*sugar under a different name*) which is in Beer. (*Hence....* Beer Belly) The next biggest insulin stimulating carb is " anything white ", including white breads, cakes, cookies, pastries, white pastas, sucrose, glucose, maltodextrin, (*more names for sugar*) then potatoes, white rice, corn, pretzels. (*not necessarily in the order I gave them to you*) (*you are getting closer to knowing why I named the book No White Diet*)

To delay the sugar being absorbed into our body we need to eat fiber and a little protein with our carbs.

There is a numerical value put on all foods. This numeral value (from 1 to 100) is known as the Glycemic Index. We are going to look into the Glycemic Index in the next chapter.

What is the Glycemic Index?

Although you might think so, all carbohydrate foods are not created equal. In fact they all behave differently in our digestive system. The glycemic index describes this difference by listing carbohydrates according to their effect on our blood glucose levels. Choosing low glycemic carbs, the ones that produce small variations in our blood glucose and insulin levels, is one of the secrets to getting the weight off and one of the keys to keeping it off.

The glycemic index is an arrangement of carbohydrates using a scale from 0 to 100 according to the span in which they raise blood sugar levels after eating. Foods with a high glycemic index are rapidly digested and absorbed resulting in a wide fluctuation of blood sugar levels. Low glycemic index foods, because they are digested slower and absorbed into the blood slower, produce a gradual rise in blood sugar and insulin levels.

Eating a lot of high glycemic foods can be damaging to your health because it pushes your body to extremes. This is especially true if you are overweight and not very active. Switching to eating mostly low glycemic carbs that slowly allow glucose into your blood stream keeps:

a.) Your energy levels balanced.

b.) You feeling fuller for longer between each meal.

c.) You're craving for food diminishing.

A low glycemic diet will help you lose and control weight. It will increase your body's sensitivity to insulin, improve diabetes control, reduce you're risk of heart disease, reduce you're blood cholesterol level, and even help prolong your endurance level. (*Pretty good Huh!*)

I am explaining the above for your information only. Do you need to carry around a book showing all the glycemic food numbers so you can pick out the right food for the next meal? NO, but if you want to you can go to glycemicindex.com and find out the glycemic number for just about any food on the market. It does get a little complicated as you have to enter each food separately.

In the meantime I want you to have an idea of what foods are high on the glycemic index and which are low. Foods containing little or no carbohydrates (such as meat, fish, eggs, wine, spirits, and most vegetables) cannot have a glycemic index value. Look at the table below to get an idea of which foods should be ingested. Don't forget that the lower the number the slower it digests. The higher the number the faster it digests. Slower is better. Low number is good. High number is bad.

Bakery, Breads	GI	Breakfast Cereals	GI
Sponge Cake	66	Rice Bran	27
Mixed Grain Bread	69	All Bran	60
Pumpernickel	71	Special K	77
White Pita	82	Kellogg's Smacks	78
Danish	84	Kellogg Mini Wheats	81
Muffin	88	Bran Chex	83
Angel Food Cake	95	Kellogg's Just Right	84
Whole Wheat Bread	99	Grape Nuts	96
White Bread	101	Shredded Wheat	99
Bagel, plain	103	Puffed Wheat	105
Kaiser Roll	104	Cheerios	106
Graham Crackers	106	Corn Bran	107
Doughnut	108	Total	109
Waffles	109	Rice Krispies	117
Vanilla Wafers	110	Corn Chex	118
Biscotti	113	Corn Flakes	119
French Baguette	136	Rice Chex	127

Rice	GI	Crackers	GI
Wild Rice, long grained	54	Soda Crackers	74
Brown Rice	66	Wheat Thins	96
White Rice, long grained	80	Rice Cakes	110

Pasta	GI	Potatoes	GI
Whole Grain Spaghetti	50	Sweet Potato	63
Multi Grain Spaghetti	55	Yams	73
White Spaghetti	60	Mashed Potato	101
White Linguine	65	French Fries	107
Gnocchi	95	Baked Potato, white	158

Fruits	GI	Vegetables	GI
Cherries	32	Artichoke, Asparagus	<15
Apple	34	Broccoli, Cauliflower	<15
Peach	40	Celery, Cucumbers	<15
Orange	47	Lettuce, Mushrooms	<15
Grapes	62	Peppers, Snow Peas	20
Raisins	64	Tomatoes	23
Banana	89	Green Peas	68
Pineapple	94	Sweet Corn	78
Watermelon	103	Pumpkin	107

Dairy	GI	Beans, Peas	GI
Whole Milk	39	Kidney Beans, boiled	42
Fat Free Milk	45	Chick Peas	47
Low Fat Yogurt, fruit	47	Black Eyed Peas	59
Low Fat Ice Cream	71	Canned Kidney Beans	74
Ice Cream	87	Fava Beans	113

Snack Foods	GI	Candy	GI
Peanuts	21	M & M's Peanut	46
Potato Chips	77	Snickers Bar	57
Popcorn	79	Chocolate Bar, 1.5 oz	70
Corn Chips	105	Life Savers	100
Pretzels	116	Jelly Beans	114

Why do I have the Craving to Eat

This is a complicated question and I will try my best to simplify it. In real simple terms, ' Low Blood Sugar ' (hypoglycemia). Let me give you an example: Everyday around 4 pm I am starving, I mean I could eat the proverbial Horse. What is happening? My body detected that the level of Glucose (sugar) in my blood is too low. It told my brain that I needed a Carb fix. My brain *(stupid that it is)* said open mouth and insert. What I did was shove anything in there that I could grab.

Technically, here is what's happening. *(Remember this because it's important.)* Our whole concept with this lifestyle of eating is to slow down the ingestion of sugar. When sugar is absorbed slowly the rise in blood sugar is slowed, the insulin (produced by the pancreas) is injected slower and the drop of blood sugar is slowed. This slow drop of blood sugar translates into less cravings for carbohydrates. *(viscous circle but that's how it works)*

Let me explain it another way. When you eat a lot of High Carb (sugar) foods, foods with a high glycemic index. The pancreas says " We need insulin to stop the sugar." The pancreas responds and gives us a dose of insulin. Usually it does to good of a job giving us plenty of insulin. The blood sugar drops like a stone and you have another craving for food.

Bottom line: slow down the intake of sugar and you slow down the cravings to eat.

How do we do this? We eat the right foods the right way and you will see your cravings slow to a manageable level.

Stay away from These Items

I want you to put the next 5 items in your memory banks. Don't forget them as they are your key to getting to a satisfactory body weight. Stay away in the order I give them to you.

Sugar
Enriched Flour (white)
Animal Fats, especially pork and beef
Hydrogenated Oils/ Trans fats
Syrups

Now, lets talk about each one. Let me be a little technical. This is important but it's not so important that you absolutely have to know it. If you don't like my discussion go on to the next chapter.

Sugar:
Sugar acts as a stimulus in causing our pancreas gland to secrete one of the bodies most powerful hormones, Insulin! Insulin does have some good effects such as regulating our blood sugar level but insulin also causes our bodies to store excess sugar as fat. It also stops the previously stored fat from breaking down and insulin signals our livers to make cholesterol. Be sure to stay away from Sugar that is spelled Maltose or Sucrose, Lactose and Fructose. All are Sugar

Enriched Flour: Enriching flour is necessary because the processing used to make white flour destroys some of the nutrients that were originally present in the whole grain. I am now going to quote Dr. Oz.*(Dr. Mehmet Oz is perhaps the most accomplished and respected cardiothoracic surgeon in the United States.)* "The reason they enrich it is because they already stripped out anything that was worth a darn in it, and they add a little bit back so it doesn't look so bad."

Animal Fats: Animal fats are fats obtained from animal sources. Animal fats are often claimed to be unhealthy due to their association with high cholesterol levels in the blood. Animal fat contains some cholesterol, but saturated fat (a large component of animal fat) stimulates cholesterol production in humans and so animal fat contributes to high cholesterol levels.

Hydrogenated Oils: I can go on and on about Trans Fats and Hydrogenated Oils. This is going to be a quick course. An example of one of the first hydrogenated oil is Crisco, which was patented in 1911. It's a combination of palm and cottonseed oil mixed with Lard and animal fats. Technically, during the process of hydrogenation, hydrogen atoms are moved to what is called the opposite side of the double bond of the molecular structure of the fatty acid in the oil. This newly formed molecular configuration of the fatty acid has been named "trans", meaning "on the other side of." Trans-fatty acids alter the normal transport of minerals and other nutrients across cell membranes. It weakens the protective structure and function of the cell. To make it, Hydrogenation gas is fused into the oils using a metal catalyst, aluminum, cobalt, and nickel. Without the metals, the hydrogen could not be fused into the oils. All are toxic metals to the body. This fusion takes place under pressure at temperatures of 248-410 degrees. In other words, the oils are changed molecularly. When you compare this changed essential fatty acid, which has now become a trans- fatty acid, it matches the same molecular structure of Stearic Acid. One of the uses of Stearic Acid is in the making of candles. It makes candles hard. Could this have the same affect on the human body in the form of hardening of arteries? *(Too technical, HUH ? I'm sorry but it was necessary to explain what it means.)*

In simpler terms, hydrogenated fats are solid at room temperature, e.g.. Lard. Think about the roast you had for dinner. After eating and during clean up- you see large areas of solidified white fat that sticks to the dish. *(yuk)*

In addition to all of the above, by hydrogenating oils, more volume is produced. It increases the volume of the oil thus making more available to be sold. *(we capitalists call this increasing profits)*

Syrups: In cooking, a syrup is a thick, viscous liquid, containing a large amount of dissolved sugars. *(Remember what I said about Sugar?)* The viscosity (thickness) arises from the multiple hydrogen bonds between the dissolved sugar and the water. Example: Artificial maple syrup is made with water and an extremely large amount of dissolved sugar. The solution is heated so more sugar can be put in than normally possible

Exercise, did you say Exercise ?

No, I did not say you have to exercise. In the first chapter called 'Let's be Honest' I told you that it is not necessary to exercise. Well...................... it's not necessary but it sure will help. *(OK, OK, OK stop swinging that bat at me, I really didn't mean it.)* Remember this fact: Muscles burn calories 45 to 50 times faster then Fat does. More muscle, faster weight loss.

Let's talk about this a little bit before you become rash over the subject. *(I hate it when people get violent.)* Before you start any exercise program you need to talk to your Doctor. I exercise 5 days a week. All 5 days I do at least 30 minutes in the Zone. (heart rate zone) I usually do an hour. Three of the 5 days I include some strength exercises. *(disgusting, Huh ?)* Were not looking for Navy Seals here. I am just asking for a little exercise each day.

My suggestion to you is to go out and buy a Heart Rate Monitor. It's a little watch-like item you put on your wrist and a band around your chest that sends your heart rate to the watch. The watch has a timer and an alarm that tells you if you are in or out of the Zone.

What's the Zone? The zone is where your body burns fat calories. If your heart rate is too low you are burning calories at such a slow rate that your not accomplishing anything. If your heart rate is too high then you're burning sugar and not some of that fat we all want to burn. You can buy a heart rate monitor for under $100.00. I have a Polar like the one pictured to the right. You can find this on the internet at polarusa.com.

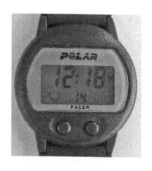

There are 3 key target zones that help you achieve the goals you want.
60-70% Lose Weight
70-80% Improve Aerobic Fitness
80+ %   Increase Athletic Performance
If you want an exact estimate of your zone you can go to polarusa.com on the web and click on Resource Center, then follow the instructions.
How do I find my *Zone ?* A quick formula is to subtract your age from 220 and multiply this number by .60 for the low range of 60% or by .70 for the range of 70% Example: You're 60 years old: you subtract 60 from

220 which equals 160, then 160 times .70 which equals 112. Or 112 heartbeats per minute. Keep your heart rate there for 70%, which is the top of your lose weight zone. You can also use the following chart to find your zone. To find your target heart rate locate your age category down the left side and find the heartbeats per 10 seconds under the 60% and 70% section of the chart. Then take this figure times 6. This is your fat burning heart rate zone.

Example: You are 45 years old, looking to the right you see that under 60% your heart rate should be 18 beats for 10 seconds and under 70% your heart rate should be 20 beats for 10 seconds. 18 x 6 = 108 or 108 beats per minute. 20 x 6 = 120 or 120 beats per minute. Your zone for losing fat is between 108 and 120 beats per minute.

Finding your pulse is simple if you don't have a heart rate monitor. The easiest way to find your pulse is to place the index and middle fingers gently on the side of the neck, next to the throat or with hands palm up press two fingers of the opposite hand on the outer wrist region just before the hand begins.

AGE	55%	60%	70%	80%
20	19	21	24	27
25	18	19	23	26
30	17	19	22	25
35	17	19	22	25
40	17	18	21	24
45	16	18	20	23
50	16	17	20	23
55	15	17	19	22
60	15	16	19	21
65	14	16	18	21
70	14	15	18	20
75	13	15	17	19

We are interested in the middle Zones, 60% to 70% of your heart rate. Put on the heart rate monitor and go out and walk a bit. You will be able to be in the zone with just a little effort. I would like to see you walk at least 30 minutes 5 days a week staying in the Zone. I can tell you after 5 years I still walk and stay in the zone. (*Besides.....I have a tough wife that beats me if I don't do it.*) Don't believe those people that say you have to jog all the time. Jogging is not, I repeat NOT good for you. (*To hard on our fat bones and joints*)

On three of the 5 days I would like to see you do some strength exercise. Why?.... Because building muscles is beneficial. Muscles burn more calories then fat does. I use a Total Gym which is inexpensive and lets you do about anything you want to do (totalgym.com) I also do crunches, yes.. sit-ups. *(Crazy Huh ?)* I have found that the exercising really helps take the pounds off. Besides, it's great to not ' huff and puff ' every time I try to do anything. I see my friends really perspiring and puffing, at the slightest exertion while I am not even breathing hard.

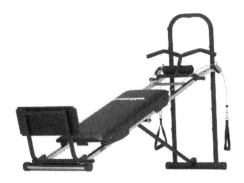

If you can't do the above because your too lazy or want to use that " I just don't have the time" excuse, at least do some exercise besides bringing the fork to your mouth. How about some simple things like parking your car at the furthest parking place in the Mall or grocery store instead of the nearest parking place to the door. If you're in an apartment house use the stairs instead of the elevator. Take it easy at first, rest when necessary. Soon you will see that you're climbing those stairs like Rocky. *(YES !)*

One more thing, Quit Smoking

I am not going to get into a discussion about this one. Just quit, I don't care how or why or what your excuses are, just quit. Use any means you can.

You know it's bad for you. I know it's bad for you.

' Quit.'

People say that "quitting is going to make me gain weight". My answer to that is I quit 26 years ago and didn't gain an ounce.(*I didn't lose any either*) My secret *(coming from a friend of mine)* was to chew a stick of sugar free gum or suck on a mint candy each time I had the urge. *(Let me tell you I had pockets full of candy and gum)*. Luckily, my dentist turned me on to sugar free candy. The urge went away after a couple of weeks.(*or was it months.*) My wife was happy because she didn't have to carry around a spare pack of cigarettes or a lighter. *(she never smoked)*

Do I still get the urge, No. The other day when I was a bit stressed *(actually a lot stressed)* over a situation I did notice myself reaching for my shirt pocket where I carried my cigarettes. Strange, Huh ?

Before we tell you What to Eat, Lets look at Labels

I have a bad habit (*actually I have many*). When I walk into a grocery store I look to see what people are putting in their baskets. (*Tacky, Huh ?*) I am amazed at what people buy and eventually eat. No one seems to look at the labels. Even our congress got smart (*isn't that amazing*) and passed laws to inform you as to exactly what is in the foods we eat. Then I realized that nobody has ever taught people how to buy or how to decipher these labels that the government so nicely placed upon our food. Well............... here I am to teach you just how to read the labels and which food to buy, or I should say which food not to buy.

Rule #2 Read the Labels before you buy.

You need to start learning this. No....... You have to learn this. I am not going to bore you. (*Well, maybe a little.*)

Here is a photo of the Nutrition Facts portion of the Label from a package of low fat Lunch Meat. I am going to give you a long explanation of the label (one time) because you need to know this stuff really well.... Then we will take a short look and show you quickly how to pick your foods. Some nutritionists will say you need to know everything on the label. I disagree, after all... are you going to spend 3 hours every week looking at labels in the grocery store?

It's really pretty simple so lets look together. All the Nutritional Labels

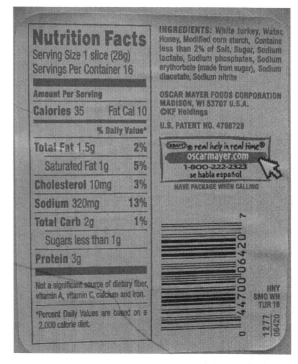

are about the same whether it's on a piece of meat or a box of cereal. Lets take a label from a package of Lunch meat first. This is a package of Oscar Meyer Lean White Turkey, honey smoked, 95% Fat Free. You will notice the Nutrition Facts are on the back of this package. Sometimes they are on the front or side. Just hunt around, you'll find it.

First is **Serving Size**: Right underneath Nutrition Facts. This label says 1 serving is 1 slice. (*Who are they kidding? they expect me to eat one thin slice of this and be happy?*) Of course not, the government says this is the way they must list the information. I want to warn you now that a serving size is not necessarily logical.

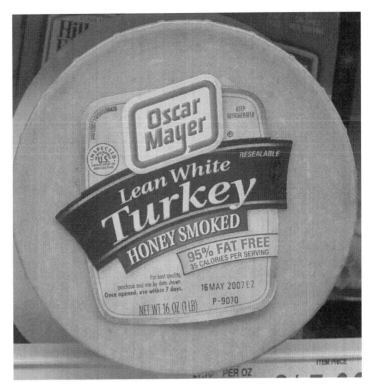

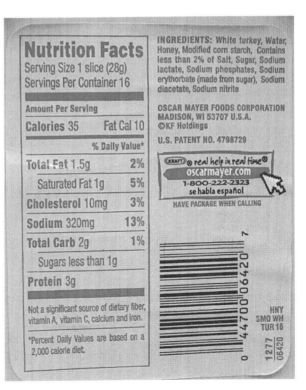

Nutrition Facts

Serving Size 1 slice (28g)
Servings Per Container 16

Amount Per Serving

Calories 35	Fat Cal 10

% Daily Value*

Total Fat 1.5g	2%
Saturated Fat 1g	5%
Cholesterol 10mg	3%
Sodium 320mg	13%
Total Carb 2g	1%
Sugars less than 1g	
Protein 3g	

Not a significant source of dietary fiber, vitamin A, vitamin C, calcium and iron.

*Percent Daily Values are based on a 2,000 calorie diet.

INGREDIENTS: White turkey, Water, Honey, Modified corn starch, Contains less than 2% of Salt, Sugar, Sodium lactate, Sodium phosphates, Sodium erythorbate (made from sugar), Sodium diacetate, Sodium nitrite

OSCAR MAYER FOODS CORPORATION
MADISON, WI 53707 U.S.A.
©KF Holdings

U.S. PATENT NO. 4798729

real help in real time
oscarmayer.com
1-800-222-2323
se habla español
HAVE PACKAGE WHEN CALLING

HNY
SMO WH
TUR 16

1277
06420

Some labels show a serving size as an unrealistic value just as a trick to have the label info not look so bad.

You need to understand that if your having 4 slices then your having 4 servings accordingly which means 4 times the calories and 4 times the fat calories listed on the label.

Servings per container: This explains how many slices are in the container. This package has 16 servings or 16 slices of lunch meat.

Now comes the important stuff.

Amount per Serving: the following explains how many Total Calories and how many Calories are from Fat in 1 slice of this product. (one serving)

Calories: 35   Fat Cal: 10

This is good, the Fat Calories ideally should be less then 33% of the total calories. It is very important to look at the label, go immediately to Calories and Fat Calories and if it has more then 1/3rd Fat Calories (33%) in a portion, you might decide to put the product back on the shelf.

Total Fat: 1.5 grams,*(by the way, there are 9 calories in every gram of fat).* This tells you that one slice gives you 2% of the total fat you are to have in one day based on a 2000 calorie a day diet. *Let me tell you that if you have 50 slices of this in one day (which would be 100% of what you could have) you would be a rollin down the isles and not walking down them.*

Saturated Fat: 1 Gram or 5%. 20 slices would give you 100% of what you are allowed.

Cholesterol: 10 milli grams or 3% of the maximum of what you should have in one day.

Sodium: 320 grams or 13% of the maximum of what you should have.

Total Carb : 1% of the total carbohydrates you should have in one day.

Sugars: less than 1 gram. Good, very good, stay away from sugars!

Protein: 3 grams . You need protein, it's good for you

Ingredients: I could go through the list and explain everything bad but instead I want to tell you to always look at the first 4 or 5 items and remember that the largest ingredient is listed first, second largest ingredient is listed second etc. Let's look at the ingredients: White Turkey, (good), Water (good) Honey (not so good, contains sugar), Modified Corn Starch (not so good). "Contains less then 2%." Everything after that states less then 2 % which is just not worth discussing it's such a small amount. Salt is OK but not great as it tends to raise blood pressure and it holds water.

Lets take a short look at the Label. This is what you are going to do in the store. After all, you don't want everyone walking down the isles staring at this crazy person blocking the isle while their reading 'No White Diet'. Besides, it would take you 3 hours to read the labels and 30 minutes to shop the store. Pick up the package and look for the label. (*Believe me it's there, it's just that they want to hide it especially if it contains items you shouldn't eat.*) First, look at the **Calories** and **Calories from Fat** or **Fat Calories**. If the Fat Calories are less then 40% of the total calories it's worth looking further. If NOT, PUT it BACK on the SHELF. This label says Calories 35 and 10 calories from fat. Less then 30% are from fat. Very good, I would buy it.

Next look at the ingredients. Is sugar or syrups in the first 4 items. If so Put it back.

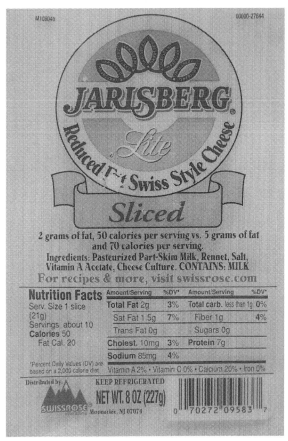

Heres a package of Jarlsberg *Lite* Reduced Fat Swiss Cheese. (*Please always buy reduced fat cheese.*) There are numerous low fat cheeses out on the market. The label describes one serving has 2 grams of fat *(18 fat calories)* and 50 total calories compared to the regular Jarlsberg cheese (from the same manufacturer) which has 5 grams of fat *(54 fat calories)* and 70 total calories per serving. I like this particular brand because it tastes very good yet it is low in fat and calories.

Take a close look at the label.
Serving Size: 1 slice.
Calories: 50, so that

Nutrition Facts	Amount/Serving	%DV*	Amount/Serving	%DV*
Serv. Size 1 slice (21g) Servings about 10	Total Fat 2g	3%	Total carb. less than 1g	0%
	Sat Fat 1.5g	7%	Fiber 1g	4%
Calories 50	Trans Fat 0g		Sugars 0g	
Fat Cal. 20	Cholest. 10mg	3%	Protein 7g	
	Sodium 85mg	4%		
*Percent Daily Values (DV) are based on a 2,000 calorie diet.	Vitamin A 2% • Vitamin C 0% • Calcium 20% • Iron 0%			
Distributed by: A	KEEP REFRIGERATED			

is 50 calories per slice. **Fat Calories:** 20, we divide that quickly in our head and we see that it's less then 50% calories from fat. Not in that 33% range I like to see but pretty good for cheese.

I have found some cheeses with a ratio lower then this but the taste was affected. I prefer to eat less of the item and continue to have the good taste.

Lets put in the cart.

This is a package of Tavern Ham from the Deli at Publix Food Stores. They slice this fresh and package it, placing it across from the Deli in a refrigerated Case. They say it's very low in fat. Let's take a look and see if we want to put it in our cart. It states to the right of the nutritional facts that this is cured with water and has less then 2% of extra ingredients like salt and sugar.

A close up of the label describes the serving size as one slice. The important part is next.
Calories: 80
Calories from Fat: 25
Less then 1/3 rd fat. This is very good.

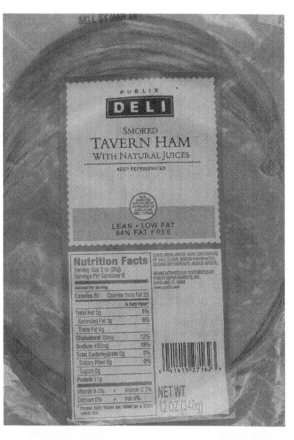

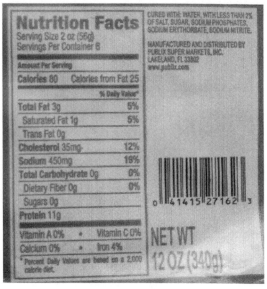

Lets put this in the cart.

See how fast you can look at the labels?

Let me show you a package of regular lunch meat so you can see the difference between the amount of Calories compared to Fat Calories. This package is also from Oscar Mayer. A typical product you or I would pick up in the store, especially for kids.

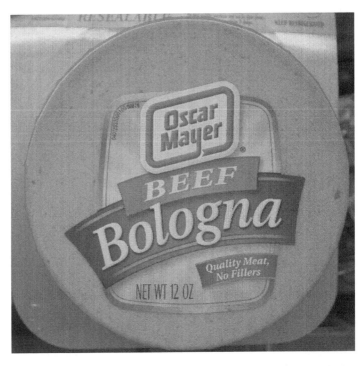

Looking at the Nutrition Facts located on the back of the package we notice that the Serving size is still one slice. The **Calories:** 90 **Fat Calories:** 70 This gives us a fat ratio of over 66% in fat, compared to 30% in fat with the previous lunch meats I presented to you.

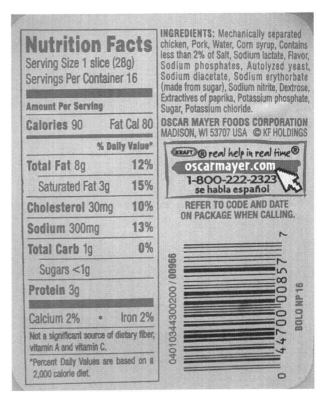

Nutrition Facts

Serving Size 1 slice (28g)
Servings Per Container 16

Amount Per Serving

Calories 90	Fat Cal 80	
		% Daily Value*
Total Fat 8g		12%
Saturated Fat 3g		15%
Cholesterol 30mg		10%
Sodium 300mg		13%
Total Carb 1g		0%
Sugars <1g		
Protein 3g		

Calcium 2% • Iron 2%

Not a significant source of dietary fiber, vitamin A and vitamin C.

*Percent Daily Values are based on a 2,000 calorie diet.

INGREDIENTS: Mechanically separated chicken, Pork, Water, Corn syrup, Contains less than 2% of Salt, Sodium lactate, Flavor, Sodium phosphates, Autolyzed yeast, Sodium diacetate, Sodium erythorbate (made from sugar), Sodium nitrite, Dextrose, Extractives of paprika, Potassium phosphate, Sugar, Potassium chloride.

OSCAR MAYER FOODS CORPORATION
MADISON, WI 53707 USA © KF HOLDINGS

KRAFT ® real help in real time®
oscarmayer.com
1-800-222-2323
se habla español

REFER TO CODE AND DATE ON PACKAGE WHEN CALLING.

Which one would you buy? (*I hope you said, "not this one."*)

If you look closely at the ingredients to the right of the Nutrition Facts you will notice that the third item in the list is corn syrup, (sugar). Remember what I said previously. If it has sugar in the first 4 or 5 items you do not want to eat it.

Now lets look at a Box of Whole Grain Cereal. I am not going to go through this slow because you would stop listening to me if I kept boring you. Lets look at it fast.

Calories: 110
Fat Calories: 15.
WOW ! Looks good HUH! With Skim Milk added there are only 150 Calories and still 15 Calories from Fat.

Without looking any further drop down to the Ingredients: Don't forget the first 4 or 5 are critical. Remember that the largest ingredient is first, next largest ingredient is second etc. The first item is Whole Grain Oats, second is sugar then corn starch, honey, brown sugar syrup. (*2nd, 3rd , 4th and 5th item is sugar*) This is NOT what you want in your body.

If you had a cup of it with Skim Milk you would only be eating 150 calories. Less then 10% of it Fat but the sugar content is

Nutrition Facts

Serving Size ¾ cup (28g)
Servings Per Container about 14

	Honey Nut Cheerios	with ½ cup skim milk
Amount Per Serving		
Calories	110	150
Calories from Fat	15	15
	% Daily Value**	
Total Fat 1.5g*	**2%**	**3%**
Saturated Fat 0g	**0%**	**0%**
Trans Fat 0g		
Polyunsaturated Fat 0.5g		
Monounsaturated Fat 0.5g		
Cholesterol 0mg	**0%**	**1%**
Sodium 190mg	**8%**	**11%**
Potassium 115mg	**3%**	**9%**
Total Carbohydrate 22g	**7%**	**9%**
Dietary Fiber 2g	**8%**	**8%**
Soluble Fiber less than 1g		
Sugars 9g		
Other Carbohydrate 11g		
Protein 3g		

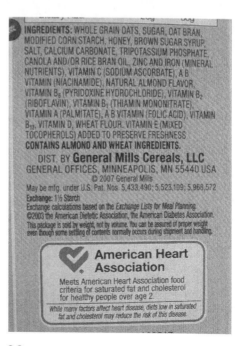

INGREDIENTS: WHOLE GRAIN OATS, SUGAR, OAT BRAN, MODIFIED CORN STARCH, HONEY, BROWN SUGAR SYRUP, SALT, CALCIUM CARBONATE, TRIPOTASSIUM PHOSPHATE, CANOLA AND/OR RICE BRAN OIL, ZINC AND IRON (MINERAL NUTRIENTS), VITAMIN C (SODIUM ASCORBATE), A B VITAMIN (NIACINAMIDE), NATURAL ALMOND FLAVOR, VITAMIN B₆ (PYRIDOXINE HYDROCHLORIDE), VITAMIN B₂ (RIBOFLAVIN), VITAMIN B₁ (THIAMIN MONONITRATE), VITAMIN A (PALMITATE), A B VITAMIN (FOLIC ACID), VITAMIN B₁₂, VITAMIN D, WHEAT FLOUR, VITAMIN E (MIXED TOCOPHEROLS) ADDED TO PRESERVE FRESHNESS. CONTAINS ALMOND AND WHEAT INGREDIENTS.
DIST. BY **General Mills Cereals, LLC**
GENERAL OFFICES, MINNEAPOLIS, MN 55440 USA
© 2007 General Mills
May be mfg. under U.S. Pat. Nos. 5,433,490; 5,523,109; 5,968,572
Exchange: 1½ Starch
Exchange calculations based on the Exchange Lists for Meal Planning. ©2003 the American Dietetic Association, the American Diabetes Association. This package is sold by weight, not by volume. You can be assured of proper weight even though some settling of contents normally occurs during shipment and handling.

♥ **American Heart Association**
Meets American Heart Association food criteria for saturated fat and cholesterol for healthy people over age 2.
While many factors affect heart disease, diets low in saturated fat and cholesterol may reduce the risk of this disease.

overwhelming. Your insulin would go crazy trying to keep up. Maybe the American Heart Association stamps their approval on this Honey Nut Cheerios product but I certainly do not.

Bottom line: You have to eat something for breakfast. Let's look for a cereal that is low in calories, fat and sugar.

Here is a box of Kashi Go Lean Crunch. Notice on the box it says Naturally Sweetened Multigrain clusters. They are telling you that they do not use sugar to make it taste better. You're probably asking right now, "does it taste good?" Well, it doesn't taste like sugar pops but I think it tastes good and it's good for you. Your next question is "how do we make it taste good?" That is pretty easy, although it has some fruit in it, lets put more on top, like maybe some fresh blueberries or raspberries or strawberries. If you really want sweet sprinkle a package of Equal or Sweet and Low over the top.

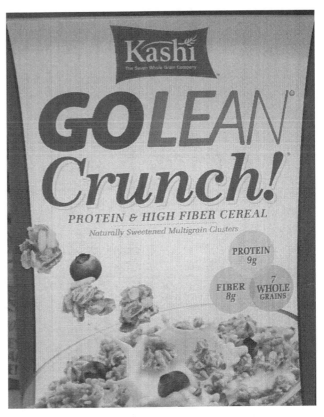

Nutrition Facts

Serving Size 1 cup (52g/1.8 oz.)
Servings Per Container About 8

Amount Per Serving	
Calories 140	Calories from Fat 10

	% Daily Value**
Total Fat 1g*	2%
Saturated Fat 0g	0%
Trans Fat 0g	
Cholesterol 0mg	0%
Sodium 85mg	4%
Potassium 480mg	14%
Total Carbohydrate 30g	10%
Dietary Fiber 10g	40%
Soluble Fiber 1g	
Insoluble Fiber 9g	
Sugars 6g	
Protein 13g	20%

Look at the Nutritional Facts,
Calories: 140
Fat Calories: 10

Are you asking " well…. it has more calories then the previous box of cereal he showed me." Actually is doesn't. Look at the serving size. This cereal serving size is 1 cup. The Cheerios I mentioned previously had a serving size of only ¾ cup. Now take a look at the

INGREDIENTS: Kashi Seven Whole Grains & Sesame® Blend (Whole: Hard Red Winter Wheat, Long Grain Brown Rice, Oats, Triticale, Barley, Rye, Buckwheat, Sesame Seeds), Evaporated Cane Juice Crystals, Soy Protein Concentrate, Brown Rice Syrup, Chicory Root Fiber, Almonds, Whole Oats, Whole Flaxseed, Expeller Pressed Canola Oil, Honey, Salt, Natural Flavor, Mixed Tocopherols (Natural Vitamin E) for Freshness.
CONTAINS WHEAT, SOY AND ALMOND INGREDIENTS.

ingredients. The first through seventh ingredients are whole oats, long grain brown rice, rye, hard red winter wheat, triticale, buckwheat, barley and sesame seeds. No Sugar.

This is much better for you, let's put this in the cart.

We're going to go shopping in the store later and really have some fun. (*Be sure to take this book with you so you really look like a nut case.*) (*You should have been with me when I was researching this book. I was running around the store with a camera taking pictures of labels. OH BOY!*)

Cleaning out the Pantry

Now that you know what to stay away from and you know that you need to exercise, lets combine the two and clean out the Pantry and Refrigerator of all those unwanted items. *What Fun !.*

While you're at it read all the labels. (it will give you good practice for the grocery store) Lets get rid of everything that has sugar in it , everything fried (including your favorite potato chips, cheese curls, fritos and pretzels) and everything higher then 50% in Fat calories.

I know, I know, your going to say "maybe I can eat it and start the diet when I'm done". Or, "it's a shame to throw away good food." So................. don't throw it away. Give it to your neighbor, one of those thin neighbors that doesn't need to lose weight, or maybe you can trade for some food you want.

You could always have a party and get rid of it quick. Invite me and maybe I can show you how to make some of it lower in fat and sugar. *(good excuse to invite me, anyway.)*

You can give it to one of the fat neighbors like me, if you like. I won't tell anyone how mean you are. How about we give the food to the local shelter for homeless people. Maybe giving it to the Church and they can have a party.

I really don't care what you do with it , just get rid of it. Come on, Come on, no better time then the present. You can read the rest of this book later. Now , it's time to Clean. If it's in the house you will eat it. No one knows better then me. I'm the fat one , Remember ?

The Do's and Don't for the first Month

Let me reiterate that this is not really a diet but a life style change. You have got to be willing to change your eating habits. You will eat tasty food, and even fast food and you will not be hungry all the time but you WILL change your life style. (*Wait till you see my recipes ! Deeeeelicious*)

For the first month you are not going to think I am the greatest guy on the planet: (*your going to love me later because I am going to give you back some of the foods you love*) I must get you back on track with your digestive system working properly. I must also get rid of your insulin resistance.(*if you are so inclined*) I am going to give you the foods you cannot eat and the foods you can eat. First the can not's. Read the list below and study it. Don't vary from it. Stay with it. You can do it, I did.
NO CHEATING

Rule #3 " Don't eat it if it's White"

Foods you CANNOT eat in the first month:
NO White Breads
NO Pastries or baked goods. (*That means No Donuts either*)
NO White Pasta. Only whole grain, whole wheat or multi grain.
NO White Rice
NO White Potatoes
NO Carrots, beets, parsnips or corn (including Popcorn, or Corn meal)
NO Candy
NO Sugar (any way shape of form) Please, Please, no Sugar.
NO Fried foods
NO Milk (except 1% or Skim)
NO Fruit juice, pineapples, raisins, bananas or watermelons.
NO Alcohol especially Beer.
NO Soft drinks with sugar. Only diet colas and un-colas
NO Cereal unless it's whole bran, barley grain, all bran or wheat grain
NO Honey
If it has Sugar (Corn Syrup, Honey, Maltose, Maltodextrin, Sucrose, Lactose, Glucose or Fructose) in the first 5 items on the label, DON'T eat it. Don't get upset now, it's not as bad as it looks. And NO I am not crazy. (*Well…. maybe a little !*) There is quite a lot of food you Can eat. Look at the next page.

Foods you CAN eat:

Breads:
Pita, wheat only
Rye sourdough
White sourdough bread (*Yes, white sourdough is completely different then White Bread.*)
Rye Whole grain bread not Rye flour bread
Pumpernickel if it's whole grain. Not this colored white bread they sell.
Whole Grain bread

Cheese (low fat, NOT regular)
American
Cheddar
Feta
Mozzarella (part skim)
String Cheese
Parmesan
Ricotta
Cottage cheese, fat free or 1%
Low fat Cream cheese

Cereal:
Rice Bran
All Bran
Oatmeal, not the instant variety
Special K
Muesli, mixed with all bran or rice bran, sugar free.

Dairy
Skim or 1% Milk
Soy Milk, low fat
Yogurt, Low Fat, artificially sweetened.
Chocolate milk, artificially sweetened

Dressings:
For Salads:
Olive oil and Red wine or Balsamic Vinegar
Look in the stores for sugar free dressings, fat free.

Desserts
Hard Candies, sugar free
Jell-O, fat free- sugar free

Fudge pops without sugar
Gum, sugar free
Popsicles, sugar free
Pudding, fat free- sugar free
Yogurt, no sugar

Eggs
Whole eggs
Egg substitutes

Fruits:
Apricots if they are fresh
Apples
Berries, all types
Cherries
Dates
Grapefruits
Lemons
Limes
Mangos
Oranges
Peaches
Pears
Plantain Bananas *(and do not fry them)*
Plums
Tomatoes

Lunch meats:
All of the fat free or low fat varieties like:
Turkey breast
Boiled ham
Cooked Ham
Turkey pepperoni
Canadian bacon

Meats:
Beef, lean cuts like filet or strip steak with all fat cut off.
Ground meat (look for 5% fat or less)
Boiled ham, very lean
Veal chops and cutlets, no fat

Nuts:
All of them but just a handful per day.

Oils:
Olive
Canola
Peanut

Poultry Products:
Chicken white meat (no skin)
Turkey white meat (no skin)

Seafood:
All fish and Shellfish
They're all good for you.

Seasonings:
If they do not have any added sugar go ahead and have them.

Spreads:
The one I recommend most frequently is Smart Balance.
I Cant believe it's not butter. (better get the spray variety so you do not over due it)

Vegetables:
All except beets, corn, carrots, peas, parsnips, rutabaga, fava beans and white potatoes.

How Big should the Portions be?

The size of the portion is not as important as the type of food you are eating. Less meat, more vegetables. More fruits, less breads and pastas even if they are whole grain.

Remember the rules:
Rule #1 Keep your mouth closed. (resist the temptations.)
Rule #2 Read the labels before you Buy (and understand them)
Rule #3 Don't eat it if it's White.

I am going to give you one more rule here to help you with portion control. Drink a glass of water before you eat. Yep ! A full glass of water. When you're hungry during the day and you want a snack, before that snack drink another glass of water. Be sure to drink a full glass of water when you wake up in the morning before doing anything else. You will be very surprised how much less you will eat if you take that glass of water first. Try not to drink much when your eating, drink just before you eat and between meals. (*It's just to complicated to go into but believe me that drinking before you eat is much better then during.*)

Rule #4 Drink a glass of water before you eat anything.

Allow me to convey an example of portion size: The best way is to look at the Plate. A regular plate (10 inch) should not be overfilling or piled up into a heap. Just fill the plate until it is not flowing over. No seconds.

In between meals if you're just dying to have something, have a handful of nuts. Not two or three handfuls, not a handful where you can't fit another nut without it spilling on the floor. (*no picking off the floor*) How about some fruit, eat an apple or one of the fruits I have mentioned above and don't forget to drink that glass of water first.

Finish your last meal by 7:30 or 8 pm. Have a little dessert. No snacks after. (*I'm really being cruel aren't I ?*)

Eat breakfast in the morning, Eggs, maybe some ham, a slice of whole wheat bread. Or have some cereal but watch it here. You really need to read the cereal box. I love it when the box says a portion size is 1/2 cup.

46

Did you ever try to eat a half of a cup of cereal ? A half of a cup isn't even a handful. I can eat 4 cups without taking a breath and this is how you gain weight. Eat one cup with skim milk and some strawberries or raspberries mixed in.

For lunch my favorite is to grab one of those wraps (*I call them Tortilla wraps*) They're in all the grocery stores and come in different flavors, spinach & herb, jalapeno (*my favorite*), garlic (*Yes!*) or whole wheat. Put a couple of slices of turkey breast or lean ham in it and then two slices of cheese (low fat) some mustard and a couple of large leaves of romaine lettuce. (*OH ....YES!*)

What about Fast Food ?

Not for the first month at all. Remember Nothing White. Please understand we have to cut down on the sugar. Even if you have a salad with fat free dressing, the dressing is loaded with sugar. I need to get your digestive system in order before you go to the fat (*oops*), I meant fast food restaurants.

There are ways to eat fast food. I will never say that fast food is good for you. In a pinch you can eat it. Don't make it a habit.

I have researched most of popular fast food restaurants. In the ensuing nutritional charts I will include the least fatty and lowest sugar foods I could find. Please look at my examples after the charts to lower the calorie and fat content even more. I have also included charts of the foods I do NOT want you to eat for most of the fast food restaurants.

Note: Some of the Fast Food companies do not want to give us the calories from fat in their Nutritional information so you have to compute it yourself. To do that you need some additional information. Should you go to their websites for further information take the Total Fat in each food item in grams and multiply it times 9 to get the fat calories. Each gram of fat has 9 fat calories.

Example: Burger King gives you the Calories in a particular item, then they give you the total fat in Grams. You take the total fat in grams and multiply it times 9 to get the Fat Calories.
Whopper, Calories: 670, Total Fat, 39 grams. (multiply the 39 grams times 9) Fat Calories: 351 (*more then 50%*)

Boston Market:

Food	Calories	Fat Cal
¼ Original Rotisserie, white meat, no skin	250	80
¼ Original Rotisserie, dark meat, no skin	260	110
Roasted Turkey	180	30
Roasted Sirloin	180	30
Green Bean Casserole, side	60	20
Steamed vegetables, side	50	20
Garden fresh coleslaw, side	80	9
Caesar Salad entree w/o dressing	140	70
Market chopped salad w/o dressing	220	80
Rotisserie Chicken (3oz)	100	20

Boston Market should be on your list of fast food restaurants to frequent.

Have ¼ chicken white meat with a side of coleslaw and either a green been casserole or steamed vegetables and you're staying under 400 calories with less then 30% fat. A great dinner.

For Lunch, have one of their Caesar Salads or Market chopped salad without dressing and put some rotisserie chicken on top. For dressing use just plain vinegar and your under 350 calories with 33% fat.

For more info on boston market go to bostonmarket.com, click on restaurant menu on the left, then click on nutrition on top.

McDonalds:

Food	Calories	Fat Cal
Grilled Chicken Classic Sandwich	420	90
Grilled Snack Wrap with Honey Must.	260	80
Asian Salad w. Grilled Chicken Newmans own Low Fat Vinaigrette	340	115
Egg McMuffin	300	110
Hamburger, regular	250	80

Example: Order a premium grilled chicken classic sandwich without the sauce. Just lettuce, tomato and onion. Then take the sandwich and throw away the top half of the bread. You will lose about 100 of the above calories and 20 of the fat calories.

If you order the Egg McMuffin I suggest to ask them to cook it with no cheese and get rid of half the bread. You will lose 100 of the calories and 30 of the fat calories.

If you can eat one of those regular Hamburgers and be satisfied, good for you. I can't so I don't order them. Throw half the bun away.

Want more info about McDonalds, go to mcdonalds.com and click on Food, Nutrition & Fitness, then click on nutrition info on the left, then Nutrition facts. They do not make it easy but all the info is there.

Please do NOT eat anything from the next table. This is to show you just how many calories and fat calories are in some of McDonalds foods.

Food	Calories	Fat Cal
Double Quarter Pounder with Cheese	740	380
Large French Fry	570	270
Chicken McNuggets (10 piece)	420	220
Chocolate triple thick shake (32 oz)	1160	240

Burger King:

Food	Calories	Fat Cal
Original Chicken Sand. w/o mayo	450	153
BK Veggie Burger w/o mayo & cheese	340	72
Croissan'wich w/egg and cheese	300	153
Tendergrill Chicken Garden Salad w/ fat free ranch Dressing	300	81
Hamburger regular	290	108

Example: If you're having the original chicken Sandwich be sure you order it without sauce and get rid of half the bread. You will cut down at least 100 calories and 20 or so calories from fat.

The Tendergrill Chicken Salad is the best for you and will fill you more then the rest. The dressing does have sugar in it.

Remember to always tell the counter person, No sauce, Mayo or Cheese.

More info? Go to bk.com, type in Nutritional Facts, hit Go, then click on Nutritional Brochure. Their info has no calories from fat so you have to multiply the total fat in grams times 9 to get the fat calories in each item.

Please do NOT eat anything from the next table. This is to show you just how many calories and fat calories are in some of Burger King's food.

Food	Calories	Fat Cal
Whopper with Cheese	760	423
Triple Whopper with cheese	1230	738
Large Fries	500	252

Wendy's:

Food	Calories	Fat Cal
Ultimate Chicken Grill Sand	370	70
Mandarin Chicken Salad/ w fat free ranch dressing	250	15
Roasted turkey Swiss Frescata/ no cheese or mayo	380	100
Junior Hamburger	280	80

What I like about Wendy's (wendys.com) is the fact that they don't play any games. They give you every bit of information you need to make a informed decision as to what to eat. They even break down each item on each sandwich so you can reduce the calories or fat.

Example: Lets say you want the Chicken Grill Sandwich and you want to get rid of half the bun, take away 80 calories and 7 calories from fat. Now you have a 290 calorie sandwich with 63 calories from fat. Take half the bun from the Hamburger and you have a 210 calorie sandwich with 73 calories from fat. It just makes me want to go to Wendy's more often because they're being honest.

For More info on Wendy's go to wendys.com, click on nutrition in the center of the page then nutrition guide.

The following is NOT for you to eat. The table is provided for comparison purposes only.

Food	Calories	Fat Cal
Double Jr. Cheeseburger deluxe	460	210
10 piece nuggets	460	270
Large French Fries	540	240

Subway:

Food	Calories	Fat Cal
6" Turkey Breast & Ham, no cheese/ with whole wheat bread.	290	45
6" Sweet onion Chicken Teriyaki	370	45
Grilled Chicken Salad with Spinach / Fat Free Honey Mustard	170	25
Minestrone Soup	90	10

Example: Subway makes many sandwich's or subs with less then 6 grams of fat. If you throw half the bread away on a 6" sub you lose 100 calories and 12 fat calories. Be sure you ask for Whole Wheat bread. No sauces except for Vinegar. One of my favorites is to order a 6" sub with Turkey Breast or Turkey Breast and Ham on Whole Wheat bread, (*no cheese because their cheese is not low in fat*) then I ask for lettuce, tomato, onions, green peppers, jalapenos,(*Yes!*) black pepper, oregano and vinegar, no oil.

I have a diet soda and sit and eat only half the bread. Still fills me up, especially if I drink a glass of water before eating. Then I'm rollin out of the restaurant I'm so full and I only had 190 calories and 33 from fat. (*This is a happy puppy*)

This is another chain willing to allow the consumer to have all the nutritional information they want. Very refreshing.

For more info on Subway go to subway.com, click on Menu/Nutrition on the top and scroll down to nutrition then click on the item you want to have information on, like Sandwiches or Salads.

Quiznos:

Food	Calories	Fat Cal
Small Turkey Lite on wheat	334	54
Small Honey bourbon Chicken	359	54

The only nutritional information they will give you is for a Small Turkey Lite sandwich or a Small Honey Bourbon Chicken.

Personally I find it regrettable that Quiznos will not publish the nutritional information. I went to two of their stores and found the same attitude.

For more info go to quiznos.com, click on Menu then nutrition information. I will write them a letter of complaint. *(you should also)* Maybe we can change their ways.

Kentucky Fried Chicken:

Food	Calories	Fat Cal
Tender Roast Sandwich w/o sauce	300	40
Roasted Caesar Salad with Original Ranch Fat Free Dressing	255	80
Original Chicken Breast and Drumstick no skin or breading, side of green bean	340	120

If you really want their chicken then get an Original breast and drumstick and take off all the skin and breading, have a side of green beans. Add a house side salad with fat free ranch (*has sugar*) and the total meal is 390 calories and 120 calories from fat.

The Tender Roast Sandwich can be reduced by throwing away half the bread. To get full feeling in that tummy have a side salad with fat free ranch dressing.

For info on the Colonel go to kfc.com and click on nutrition on the top of the page. Then click on Nutrition Guide

Let's look at the problems you can get into by ordering the wrong items at KFC. Please do NOT eat any of the following.

Food	Calories	Fat Cal
3 piece Dinner extra crispy, (breast, thigh, drumstick),potato wedges, cole slaw, biscuit	1460	750
Triple crunch sandwich	640	320
Crispy Caesar Salad, ranch dressing	560	360

Pizza Hut:

Food	Calories	Fat Cal
Large Thin n Crispy veggie lovers, 2 slices	520	180
Medium Thin n Crispy Pepperoni & mushroom, 2 slices	380	140
Spaghetti w Marinara sauce, side salad w 2 tablespoon lite Italian dressing	560	117

If you insist on having their Pizza then 2 slices of the medium thin and crispy with pepperoni & mushrooms is the least calories and fat calories. They have a lite italian dressing but it still has a lot of fat calories (45) with 70 total calories.

Bottom line, try and stay away from Pizza Hut.

For more info on Pizza Hut go to pizzahut.com, click on nutrition, then scroll down to the printable nutrition guide on the bottom of the page.

The following is what NOT what you eat at Pizza hut.

Food	Calories	Fat Cal
Large Meat Lovers, pan, 2 slices	1060	560
Wings (6) with ranch dipping sauce	550	390

Dominos Pizza:

Food	Calories	Fat Cal
Large Thin crust with veggies, 2 slices	360	170
Medium Thin Crust w pepperoni & mushrooms, 2 slices	350	216
Garden Salad w light italian dressing	90	45

Dominos is about the same as Pizza Hut or any other Pizza type place. Be careful when you eat Pizza. It's high in calories and fat. Good for a splurge but not as a habit.

For more info on Dominos go to dominos.com then click on 'See the Menu' on the upper right, then under pizza on the left click on Nutritional info or click on sides etc.

I must say this is the most complicated chart I have ever seen. They really make it hard for you to compute a simple slice of Pizza. You have to add the crust, cheese, sauce, toppings separately for each slice. They could really make it easier. Let's write another letter.

Taco Bell:

Food	Calories	Fat Cal
2 Beef Crunchy Tacos, Fresco	300	140
Chicken Fiesta Burrito	340	80
Taco Salad, Fiesta with no shell	230	25

The way to keep the fat and calories down with Taco Bell is to order Fresco style. They will use Fiesta Salsa in place of the sauce or cheese.

For information go to tacobell.com, click on nutrition guide then click on printable nutrition guide or Fresco style.

Do NOT eat anything from the next table. This is to show you just how many calories and fat calories are in some of Taco Bell's food.

Food	Calories	Fat Cal
Beef & potato Burrito	540	220
Zesty Chicken Border Bowl	730	360
Nachos Bell Grande	790	390
Grilled Stuft Burrito, Beef	720	290

Dunkin Donuts:

Food	Calories	Fat Cal
Plain, Onion or Wheat Bagel w lite vegetable cream cheese	420	100
Ham, egg & cheese English Muffin	310	90
French Cruller	150	70
Strawberry, Apple Crumb, Blueberry Crumb, or Maple frosted Donut	240	90

The Egg, Ham and Cheese english muffin seems like the way to go. Personally I would tell them to eliminate the cheese and save some calories and lots of fat.

As far as Donuts go, there all pretty bad and loaded with sugar. The French Cruller and the sugar raised donut are the least with 150 calories and 70 from fat.

For more information on Dunkin Donuts go to dunkindonuts.com, click on nutrition in very small print on the upper side. Then click on printable nutrition guide.

The following is to be your NO eat list for Dunkin Donuts:

Food	Calories	Fat Cal
Sausage, Egg, Cheese Croissant	690	460
Banana Walnut Muffin	540	230
Glazed Cake Donut	350	170

The First Month is Over, Now What?

If you didn't cheat your digestive tract is probably back to where it belongs. If you did cheat, SHAME ON YOU. Go back and do another month without cheating. (*I'm cruel but honest*)

I am not going to ration you on the amounts you should eat. I expect you to eat smart. Later in this book you will get some delicious recipes to use but it's really not necessary to follow the recipes I give you.

You have to understand the 'life style', the way to eat and the types of food you can eat. We are trying to eat low fat, low sugar foods. It's basically a simple process. Listen to what I say, eat the food's I suggest and as time goes by you will lose weight. Obviously, the fewer high sugar, high fat foods you eat the more you will lose. The more of them you eat the less you lose. Eat less White foods and lose more weight.

Park that car in the furthest spot at the mall and walk the rest of the way and you will lose more weight. Get your self a heart rate monitor and walk in the Zone for at least 30 non stop minutes each day and you will lose still more. Start some strength training exercises with weights and you will lose more yet. Don't forget that muscle burns calories faster then fat does.(*up to 50 times faster*) The more muscle mass you have, the quicker you burn calories and the more weight you lose.

Foods for the Rest of Your Life

The following is a list of foods that are acceptable for the rest of your life. Follow it and stay slim. Feed it to your Husband (or Wife) and children and they will stay thin. Again, a simple way to lose weight and maintain that weight loss: Please don't diet, change your life style.

Include the foods from the previous list posted for the first month. Keep the portions to a 10" plate full and no seconds. Read the labels, again, Read the Labels, it's your best way to stay slim.

Bread:
Pita, either whole wheat or stone ground
Whole Grain Breads, no corn syrup, brown sugar, molasses or honey
Rye whole grain. Not rye flour bread
Rye Sourdough
White Sourdough Bread
Pumpernickel if it's whole grain
No white bread
No white rolls
No refined wheat bread just whole grain (sugar free)
No cookies

Cereal:
Rice Bran
All Bran
Fiber One
Kellogg's Just Right
Mini Wheats, no sugar
Oatmeal, not the instant variety
Special K
Kellogg's Smacks
Kellogg's Extra Fiber All Bran
Muesli
No Cornflakes
No cereal with sugar
No Rice Krispies
No Corn or Rice Chex

Cheese: All of the following should be Low Fat
American
Cheddar
Cottage Cheese, Fat free or 1 %
Low Fat Cream cheese
Feta
Mozzarella (part skim)
Parmesan
Provolone
String cheese
Parmesan
Ricotta
String cheese
No Camembert
No Brie
No Edam

Dairy Products:
Milk, 2% or 1% or skim
Eggs and egg substitutes
Yogurt, low fat or fat free, artificially sweetened
Soy milk, low fat
Chocolate milk, artificially sweetened
No Whole milk
No regular Soy milk
No whole Yogurt

Desserts:
Chocolate at least 60% cocoa (*be careful now, just a little*)
Ice Cream, low fat and sugar free
Yogurt, sugar free
Don't forget that Cheese makes a great dessert. Fat free of course.
Hard candies, sugar free
Jell-O, fat free, sugar free
Fudge pops without sugar
Gum, sugar free
Popsicles, sugar free
Pudding, sugar free
No Cookies
No Muffins
No regular Ice Cream
No pastries either

Dressing and Sauces:
Canola Oil
Hot Sauces, sugar free
Jalapeno sauce
Olive oil
Soy
Vinegar, white, red wine or balsamic
Look for fat free, low in sugar dressings.
Worcestershire

Drinks, Juices:
Fruit juices 100% without added sugar only
Vegetable Juice, Example: V8, 100% vegetable juice.
Colas with artificial sweeteners
Coffee, caffeine free
Tea, caffeine free

Fish:
Shellfish and any other fish you like.

Fruit:
Apples
Apricots
Berries, all types
Cantaloupes
Cherries
Dates
Grapes
Grapefruits
Honeydew Melons
Kiwis
Lemons
Limes
Mangos
Oranges
Peaches
Pears
Planton Bananas, no regular bananas
Plums
No Bananas
No Canned fruit with juice packed inside
No Pineapple
No Raisins
No Watermelon

Meats:
Lunch meats if low fat.
Beef, lean cuts, fat trimmed off.
Chicken, white or dark meat is OK, no skin. No wings and legs.
Duck, careful here no skin, trim the fat
Goose, same here, no skin, trim the fat
Lamb
Rabbit
Pork Tenderloin and Lean chops
Turkey, no skin
Veal
Venison
No Processed poultry
No Honey baked ham
No Liver
No Brisket

Nuts:
All of them but limit to a handful a day.

Pasta and Rice:
Whole grain pasta
Whole grain brown rice
Wild Rice
Multigrain Pasta, there are new ones on the market. One of my favorites is made by Barilla, called Plus.
No white pasta
No white rice

Seafood:
All fish
All shellfish

Spices:
Go ahead and indulge, spices are ok. You will see most of my recipes are loaded with spices.

Spreads:
Smart Balance
Cant believe it's not Butter
Olive oil, try just a bit on toast.
No Margarine
No Butter

Sweeteners:
A lot of the artificial sweeteners are fine. Tests have shown that Aspartame used in Splenda and Equal is not as good for you. Sweet and low is best for artificial sweeteners .

Vegetables:
Asparagus
Artichokes
Beans. If you buy in cans, no sauces like ketchup or barbecue.
Black eyed peas
Butter beans, boiled
Cabbage
Celery
Cauliflower
Chick peas
Cucumbers
Bell Peppers
Broccoli
Brussel Sprouts
Eggplant
Hearts of Palm
Lentils
Lettuce any kind
Lima beans
Mushrooms, all types
Okra
Onions
Peas
Pinto Beans
Spinach
Squash
Sweet Potatoes
Tomatoes
Turnip Greens
Yams
Zucchini
No beets,
No corn,
No carrots,
No parsnips,
No rutabaga,
No baked beans
No fava beans
No white potatoes

Foods to Stay Away From

Please do not forget the Rules:

Rule #1 Keep your mouth closed. Resist the temptations.

Rule #2 Read the labels before you Buy (and understand them)

Rule #3 Don't eat it if it's White

Rule #4 Drink a glass of water before you eat anything.

Foods you Should not eat:

In the List above under Foods for the Rest of your Life I specifically listed some of the ' no- no' foods. The following should be in your memory banks to use quickly.

NO White Breads, pastries or baked goods

NO White Pasta, only whole grain, whole wheat or multi grain.

NO White Rice

NO White Potatoes, carrots, beets, parsnips, rutabaga or corn products

NO Candy unless it is sugar free hard candy.

NO White Sugar Use sugar substitutes

NO Fried foods

NO Milk (except 1% or Skim)

NO Pineapples, raisins, bananas or watermelons.

NO Alcohol except for a glass of wine, preferably red. Especially;

NO Beer.

NO Cereal unless its whole bran, barley grain, all bran or wheat grain.

If it has Sugar (Corn Syrup, Honey, Maltose, Maltodextrin, Sucrose, Lactose, Glucose or Fructose) in the first 5 items on the label, DON'T eat it.

Let's Go Shopping

Just walking into some grocery stores can seem daunting. If you carry this book with you it will help both of us. Remember the deal, I'm going to make you happy by helping you to lose weight and your going to make me happy by selling books. *(Cool !)*

At first you will have to study every label. After a while you will know what to buy automatically. You'll be saying " those people are crazy, I'm not buying that !" or " Look at the fat in there." I hope that eventually you will be saying " Did I use to eat that…...nah….I wouldn't eat something with that much fat or sugar."

Let's go shopping. One of my favorite things to do. I ask my wife all the time if I can go shopping for her. Most of the time she says 'NO'. I believe she thinks I don't like it. *(I do)*

At the end of this section I have included some blank pages so you can jot down calories, fat calories, and sugar content on some of your favorite foods as you're going through the isles. *(What fun !)* (*I could include a pencil but I thought you might consider it to be a little much.)*

Vegetables:
If you walk into my local chain grocery store you come to the vegetable area first. Here you can splurge, just pick what you want except for avocados, pineapples, melons, bananas, white potatoes, beets, corn and carrots. Stock up on the fibers like different lettuce's including mixed greens, romaine etc. Remember we are trying to eat more fibers and less proteins and fats. No calories to speak of in most vegetables and certainly no fats.

Bakery:
The Bakery is next in my grocery store. Instead of going down the bread Isle try one of the Whole Wheat or Seven Grain Breads from the bakery. If you really have to have white bread then be sure it's Sourdough White. Forget the donuts, crawlers, bagels and especially muffins *(even the bran muffins, most are not really bran)*. When you get to the bread isle try the whole wheat english muffins or whole grain bread with no sugar added. Switch to wraps; they're available everywhere and come in various flavors

like jalapeno, garlic, and spinach. Stay away from the plain variety as the flour is white..

Lunch Meats, Cheeses:
This is where your label study in the previous chapter is going to come into play. Remember to look at the Calories and the Fat Calories. You want to be at ⅓, or less, fat calories to total calories. So 100 calories would have 33 fat calories. Keep the sugar low. Try not to buy if sugar or a surrogate sugar name is in the first 4 or 5 items of the ingredients. The lunch meats will say, 95% fat free or close to that. Be sure to look at the label, don't believe what the front of the package says. There are many tricks the companies can use to fool you. With the cheese, be sure it is Lite cheese. For sandwiches get swiss lite or american lite. I happen to like the Alpine Lite cheese.

Meats:
Please stay away from the ground meat, beef and pork for the first month. Concentrate on Chicken or Turkey (and Fish) . After that first month we will start easing our way back into beef and pork. Don't forget to buy the less then 15% and hopefully 5% fat ground meat. Pick any style of chicken or turkey you like. When you get home take the skin off all of it before cooking. If you're going to rotisserie the chicken or bake the turkey, leave the skin on but be sure not to eat it.

After the first month when you're shopping for ground meat to use in hamburgers or meat loafs get 95/5 (5% fat) ground meat. Look at the labels closely and you will see 70/ 30 (30% fat) , 85/15 (15% fat) etc. Do not buy anything but the lowest in fat. If you can't find it then ring the bell and call the butcher. He will be more then happy to get it for you. If the butcher doesn't want to help, go to another store.(*Competition is good)* For steaks, again look at the fat content, you want the leanest meat you can find. Same with roasts. I stay away from pork because it is just too high in fat.

Seafood:
Go crazy here, any fish you want and all the shell fish, it's all good for you. Look at the dinner recipes below if you want an exact match but don't forget you can substitute just about any fish with another and ac-complish the same recipe. Pick the freshest fish in the market. We hap-pen to have a great seafood section at our local store and the people be-hind the counter are always accommodating . Ask them which fish is the freshest that day.

Canned Food:
I am not a big believer in canned food, especially vegetables. The fresh vegetables are better for you.(*and taste better*) Should you decide to purchase the canned variety the following seem to be acceptable. Mushrooms, turnip greens, sauerkraut, peas, green beans, red beans, black beans, black eyed peas, chick peas, pink beans, kidney beans, lima beans, great northern beans, field peas, white beans, lentils, red kidney beans, pinto and cannellini beans. No baked beans, they're full of sugar.

Soups are just loaded with fat, sugar and very high in salt. (*helping to produce high blood pressure in many individuals*). I can't go through each one with you but studying the labels does the trick. Stay away from cream soups, look at the red or clear broth variety like vegetable or beef barley with vegetables. Pick up some chicken and beef broth for the recipes in this book. (*low sodium*) Bouillon cubes are best as they have no fat.

Canned meats like chicken breast in water is fine. Others like canned luncheon meats, corned beef or corned beef hash are not. Most of the canned fish such as pink salmon, red salmon, jack mackerel, smoked oysters, whole oysters, crabmeat, shrimp, anchovies, tuna in water and codfish are great.

Example: Take a look at Tuna fish. You will not believe the difference between the Tuna in Oil and the Tuna in water. Obviously you are going to buy the one in water.

Sauces, Dressings:
I always pick up some spaghetti sauce when I'm at the store. Nothing like a quick dish of Pasta with one of those ' star' sauces on the market. To tell you the truth some of them are pretty good. Paul Newmann has some real good ones and all the profit goes to charity. If you like the sauce a little spicy (*like I do*) then pick up a Arrabbiata. I also like a Puttanesca with olives and those little furry fish. Again, I warn you to look at the labels, some of the manufacturers put a lot of sugar in the sauce and some have ingredients with quite a bit of Fat. (*like meat*)

I have always used tomato paste to make my own sauce. (*Comes from my mother.*) Tomato paste is just concentrated tomatoes, pureed. Saute up some onions and garlic in olive oil, add a couple of cans of paste, a couple of cans of water, add some spices, thyme, basil, oregano. Then add what ever flavoring you like. Maybe a sprig of mint (*moms favorite*), anchovies, olives or all of the above. ' Wanna mak-a meat-a sauce-a,' add the meat when you saute the onions and garlic.(*use low fat ground meat*)

69

Salsas are usually ok. I even found a chili mix made by McCormick that had very little fat and hardly any sugar.

Salad Dressings are very tricky. Look at the label. If it states a specific amount of calories with no calories from fat, be careful. "Ahhhhhhh"....... you say, this is the one. NO it's not. Look at the ingredients and see how much sugar is in it. Stay away from the sugar. Better to take one with a little fat and no sugar. I found a couple made by South Beach that were very good. They make a Ranch, Italian and Balsamic that are all low in sugar and fat. Forget about mayonnaise or even miracle whip, both have lots of fat and sugar. Even the reduced fat Helmans which has 20 total calories per serving and 20 calories from fat has a lot of sugar in it. (*100% fat*)

Hot sauces, and soy sauces are all right. Teriyaki usually has a lot of sugar. I did find one made by Hokan that was acceptable. Many of the barbecue sauces have a lot of sugar in them. There is one by KC Masterpiece low cal that had only 10 calories per serving and 0 from fat. Low on sugar also. If you like barbecue sauces look further in this book under Side Dishes and Sauces and make one of my recipes. I limit the sugar and mine are very low in fat.

Pasta:
Some of you are going to have a hard time switching to whole wheat pasta. (*I did*) Since one of my staples is pasta I know how you feel. I still am not crazy about it although my wife loves it. I have found a multi grain pasta from the largest pasta maker in the world, Barilla, (called Plus) that is just delicious. I take the multigrain pasta and mix in some whole wheat pasta with it. (*stolen from my wife's pan*) We are always cooking two different pans of pasta. One for the whole wheat and one for the regular. Remember the rules, No White, so that means no white pasta.

Cereals:
Another problem area. I know most of you eat a bowl of cereal before either dashing to work or before taking the kids to school. Reeeeaaaalllly be careful here. Every box has another slogan telling you how good it is and how low in fat it is and blah, blah, blah. It would take 3 of these books just to teach you how to buy cereal. I can only say, look close at the labels. Look real close. I gave you an example under the chapter for labels. Watch out for sugar and other names they use for sugar. Buy only bran or whole grain cereals. If the taste is not what you like add some berries to the bowl. Look at my suggestions for cereal under Foods for the rest of your life.

Fruit Juices:
Forget about them, especially for the first month, just too much sugar. After the first month only 100 % fruit juice. Again, the manufacturers love to play word games on the labels. Be sure it's 100% juice. V8 100% vegetable juice had only 50 calories per serving and 0 from fat. Campbell's tomato juice was the same. Sunsweet prune, unfiltered apple juice and Oceanspray ruby red grapefruit were low in fat but high in calories per serving compared to the tomato or V8.

Pickles:
Most dill and even some bread and butter pickles are without calories or calories from fat. Relish is full of sugar so stay away from it.

Dairy Products:
Milk just has to be skim or evaporated fat free. (*good for baking recipes*) (I *think it's smart to stay away from the 1 and 2 percent variety*) For your coffee there are fat free creamers in a variety of flavors. (*my favorite is International or Carnation Hazelnut*) Buy low fat cheeses which will usually have Lite on the label.   They're ok but do not eat a lot of cheese as even the low fat varieties are still pretty high in fat. If it's mozzarella be sure it's skim and not whole milk.

Alcohol:
I am really sorry to tell you that you have to quit the Beer. Do not even think of picking up a six pack. NO, no, no.
Red wine is good and white wine is OK. The white zinfandel has more sugar compared to a dryer wine. Consequently, the dryer the better.
As far as hard liquor goes, I would say no, especially for the first month.

Soft Drinks:
Your just going to have to drink diet sodas. Way to much sugar in the regular ones. Sorry

Snacks:
Soy nuts, soy crisps and maybe Terra Chips (vegetable chips) are somewhat acceptable after the first month. Both South Beach and Zone make snack bars that are low in sugar and fat for those between meal times when your just starving. They are very good tasting. Peanut butter is not too bad if you buy only the organic type like Smuckers Organic. Pour the oil off when it separates. I like it on a stalk of celery for a snack. Look in the snack section of the recipes for more.

Sweets:
The only cake even halfway acceptable is sponge cake(angel food). Great with berries over the top. Applesauce makes a good addition to your dessert menu. Jell'o fat free is also good. For baking try Splenda sugar substitute in any baking recipe requiring sugar or Sugar Twin brown sugar (substitute) for the recipes requiring real brown sugar.

Syrup:
In the recipe section, under breakfast, I included some some pancake and waffle *(oat and whole wheat)* recipes. *(Yum!)* You are going to want to eat them with maple syrup. I found one from Log Cabin, one from Steeles and another from Cary's that were sugar free.

Pre Packaged Foods:
I think that if you want to save money and lose weight you will stay away from the prepackaged foods which are frozen and expensive. If thats what you want for an occasional meal be sure to look closely at the label and remember NO White. Most have a lot of potatoes because their inexpensive to produce. The pasta dishes are all with white pasta. Not for you. There are some produced by South Beach that are fine. (no potatoes) I also looked at items like frozen waffles, no, no, no. Even the whole wheat ones were made with mostly standard white enriched flour with just a little whole wheat flour. Stay away.

Best advice I can give you is stay away from the prepackaged foods.

Notes

Additional Information

If you would like additional information on some of the topics I have broached in this book, please go to the following websites.

To contact us go to www.nowhitediet.com, don't forget to send us some of your recipes. If you should have a favorite recipe that you feel is high in fat or sugar, send it to us and we will try to revamp it and make it lower, still retaining the taste.

To really learn how the digestive system works, go to:
http://digestive.niddk.nih.gov/ddiseases/pubs/yrdd/

To learn more about the glycemic index and how it affects your diet go to: www.glycemicindex.com

A good place to learn about healthy food is at: www.whfoods.com

For information on the Total Gym, go to: www.totalgym.com

For information about the heart rate monitor go to: www.polar.com

New Cookbook on the way

I am working on a new book, a cook and recipe book called 'An Array of Delectables '. It really started some years ago when my mother died. She was from Italy and loved to be in the kitchen. As a matter of fact I don't remember a time when she wasn't in the kitchen making food for us or my dad or even the neighbors. She even made food for the workers who took care of the street, electric poles or telephone. There would always be strangers at the table eating spaghetti and talking with mom.

Anyway, I decided to take some of her favorite recipes, combined with my wife's and make a book. After thinking about it *(one of my problems)* and writing this book I thought it would be a better book if I included other peoples recipes with a little story about them.

So…………….. how about it? Send me one or a bunch of your recipes and we will cook them up *(What Fun!)* and test them. *(I'm the tester. Do you see why I have a problem with weight?)*

Go to the website, www.nowhitediet.com, and click on contact us. There you will find our e mail address. *(It changes now and then because of spam)* If you want to send it through the US Mail use the following address:

Horizon Unlimited Inc.
819 Peacock Plaza #668
Key West, Florida 33040

No
WHITE
Diet !

Part Two

Recipes

In the first chapter , let's be honest, I mentioned the fact that during this lifestyle diet you would be eating delicious food and losing weight. The following recipes are being presented for your perusal. See exactly how well you can eat and still lose weight.

Many basic recipes are not included in the list that follows. Some of my favorite lunches or dinners are extremely simple.

I enjoy throwing a chicken breast on the Barbecue with a little squeeze of lemon and some basil on it or maybe brushing on some Teriyaki sauce instead. For a side dish, I might steam a bunch of broccoli in a sauce pan with just a little water. Cook it for 5 minutes until it turns bright green. Salt, pepper and a little Smart Balance or Can't Believe it's not Butter on top and you have a great meal.

I also enjoy having a Steak Burger (*buy less then 10% fat ground beef*) on the Bar-b with just garlic, salt & pepper for seasoning. Saute some fresh mushrooms with a tablespoon of Smart Balance or Can't Believe it's not Butter, and place it on top of the Steak Burger. On the side maybe a Sweet Potato, microwaved for 5 minutes and served with pepper and Smart Balance. If you also want a vegetable then steam some asparagus, squirt some lemon on and serve.

One of the favorites for both my wife and I is to have hamburgers with a bottle of champagne. I use the same ground beef that I do for the steak burgers with the same seasoning. I cut up some slices of tomato and onion then lay out some leaf lettuce on a dish. I love using sourdough bread which I spray with a little water and place in a hot oven (450 degrees) for 5 or 7 minutes. It makes a crunchy crust. Don't slice it the regular way but the long way. Then cut of a portion of the end for your hamburger. On the side have a salad. (*Pick one from the section on Salads*) Buy a bottle of inexpensive champagne like Andre or if you really want to splurge, a bottle of Freixenet Brut Cordon Negro in a black bottle. (*Sexy!*) (*$8.99 on sale around here.*) We always use china and linen napkins with our hamburgers. Set a flower on the table and use nice flute type champagne glasses. It's a party!

I guess what I'm saying is ' simple is good'. You don't need gourmet cooking to eat nutritious and/ or delicious food. If you desire more of the following great recipes taken from a varied number of sources, including my wife and myself, please go to our web site www.nowhitediet.com and download them. We will constantly add new recipes. *(especially if you send us some)*

We would love to hear from you with your favorite recipes. Just e mail them to us and we will publish them on the website. Be sure to let us know if we can use your name with the recipe.

Breakfast

Breakfast can sometimes be a bowl of Bran cereal and skim milk or a couple of slices of whole wheat bread. How about a whole wheat english muffin with smart balance spread on top if your in a hurry.

One simple recipe I received from my grandfather is to soft boil eggs 3 ½ minutes with a slice of rye or 7 grain bread on the side. I remember when I was young how he use to sit at the table alone with the egg in a little cup *(blue flowers on it)* and have his toast on a small plate. *(also with the same blue flowers)* A small glass *(a little bigger then a sherry glass)* of red wine, sitting just behind the egg cup, and always a white linen napkin with a small spoon in the center. He would invite me to sit with him and ask my grandmother to give me a glass of milk. I once asked him what was in the glass. He told me that it was wine, made from grapes, and that he had a small glass with every meal. My grandfather was from Italy *(he was Venetian)*. Maybe .... just maybe the Italians had a good idea with the red wine. What do you think?

All of us have different urges in the morning. For example; my wife could shred the wallpaper and eat it it like bran cereal when she first wakes up. *(mmmmm.... I wonder if that's what happened to the walls in the bedroom)* My self, on the other hand, will get up in the morning and be satisfied with a cup of coffee. *(or two or three, maybe four)* Come around or about 12 noon, the urges start to hit. I can eat constantly from then until about 10 at night. Who is right? Neither one of us, a happy medium would be in order. Everyone says, and I agree, that food in the morning is a good idea. I am just not hungry early in the morning, but I have learned to have something even if it's a piece of dry whole wheat toast. If you're just going to have a small amount early in the morning then have another slice of toast or a piece of fruit a couple of hours later so you blood sugar doesn't go haywire by the time lunch comes around.

Remember this: we want our blood sugar level to stay constant and not go from high to lows. *(or visa versa)* This is what gives you the food cravings. The more fiber you eat and the less sugar the steadier your blood sugar remains.

If you're like me then the following recipes are for your special days.

Denver Omelette

I have never understood why this omelette is called a Denver omelette, I guess it was invented in Denver. My mother always served it and she had never been to Denver nor did she know anyone from there. Normally it's made with real eggs but we're going to use Egg Beaters or an egg substitute.

Prep Time: 10 minutes
Cook Time: 10 minutes
Serves: 2

½ cup chopped Green Pepper
½ cup chopped onion (½ onion)
1 clove garlic minced
1 cup Egg Beaters or Egg Substitute. (equal to 4 eggs)
2 tablespoons skim milk
1 tablespoon olive oil
2 slices of deli ham diced
Salt and Pepper to taste

In a small 8 inch non stick frying pan add the oil and saute the onions, peppers & garlic until the onions are translucent (approx. 3 minutes). Add the deli ham, stir 1 minute then add the eggs, salt and pepper. Turn heat to low and simmer until the mixture starts separating from the side of the pan. Turn on the broiler in your oven and put the pan on the center rack and cook until brown. If you're not sure if it's done take a small knife and slice a small slit and look in the center. It should be dry.

Serve on a large plate with some sliced tomatoes on the side dribbled with a little olive oil and chopped parsley.

Whole Wheat Pancakes

These are about the most delicious whole wheat pancakes I have ever eaten. Try them and tell me what you think.

Prep Time: 15 minutes
Cook Time: 20 minutes
Servings: 28 pancakes

1 cup all-purpose flour
2 cups whole wheat flour
1 ⅓ cups dry milk powder
1 teaspoon baking powder
1 ½ teaspoons baking soda
1 teaspoon salt
¾ cup Splenda sugar substitute
4 eggs, lightly beaten
3 cups water
¼ cup smart balance , melted
3 tablespoons white vinegar

In a large bowl, sift all-purpose flour, milk powder, baking powder, baking soda and salt. Stir in whole wheat flour.

In a small bowl, combine sugar, eggs, water, butter and vinegar. Make a well in the flour mixture, and pour in the egg mixture. Mix until smooth.

Heat a lightly oiled griddle or frying pan over medium heat. Pour or scoop the batter onto the griddle, using approximately 1/4 cup for each pancake.

Cook until pancakes are golden brown on both sides; serve hot.

French Toast with Bananas

Whole wheat french toast that really tastes good while being low in calories and low in fat to boot.

Prep time: 15 minutes
Cook Time: 15 minutes
Servings: 6

½ cup Egg substitute
1 teaspoon water
1 tablespoon nonfat milk
1 teaspoon vanilla extract
1 teaspoon grated orange zest
1 pint strawberries, tops removed then sliced in half.
12 slices Whole Wheat bread in slices
¼ cup smart balance

In a medium bowl, beat together, eggs, water, milk, vanilla extract and orange zest.

Melt a small amount of smart balance in a skillet over medium heat. Dip one slice of bread in the egg and milk mixture, allowing bread to become soaked, then place in skillet.

Cook, turning once, until both sides are golden brown.

Serve using the strawberries as garnish.

Brunch Souffle

Slices of whole wheat bread layered with smoked turkey sausage, spinach and baked in a mixture of egg and milk make this a tasty casserole.

Prep time: 15 minutes
Sitting time: overnight is best
Cook Time: 45 minutes

1 pound smoked link turkey sausage, sliced
12 slices whole wheat bread
6 slices american or swiss cheese (lite)
¼ cup green onions, chopped
¼ cup green pepper, chopped
1 teaspoon dry mustard
1 10 ounce package spinach, thawed and drained
¾ cup egg substitute
2 cups skim milk
½ teaspoon salt
¼ teaspoon pepper
½ cup whole wheat breakfast flakes crushed (cereal)

Place 6 slices of bread across the bottom of an oblong or rectangle 2 quart casserole dish. Cover each slice of bread with a slice of cheese. Layer each slice of cheese with green onions, pepper, and the drained spinach, top with sliced smoked sausage. Top with the other 6 slices of bread. Slice each sandwich in half on the diagonal.

In a bowl, combine the eggs, milk, season with salt and pepper. Pour the liquid slowly over the sandwiches. Cover and let sit over night in the refrigerator.

In the morning preheat the oven to 350 degrees fahrenheit. Sprinkle the casserole with the whole wheat crushed flakes and bake for 45 minutes or until puffed and set. Let stand 10 minutes before serving.

Paul's Fritata

I have made this recipe for hundred's of people and they all love it. You can substitute the vegetables I use with others you might have in the frig.

Prep time: 10 minutes
Cook Time: 15 minutes
Serves 4

2 tablespoons olive oil
½ green pepper sliced
1 small onion chopped fairly course
½ head broccoli cut in pieces
6 or 7 slices yellow squash
4 or 5 small mushrooms sliced in half
2 cups Egg beaters or Egg substitute
¼ cup skim milk
salt & pepper to taste
⅛ teaspoon cinnamon
3 roma tomatoes sliced.

In a bowl add eggs, milk, salt & pepper and cinnamon. Whisk until smooth.

Heat a 10 inch frying pan on the stove, add olive oil then garlic, onion and green peppers, stir with high heat until onions are translucent. (about 3 minutes) add broccoli, yellow squash and mushrooms, stir for another 2 minutes, add egg mixture and turn heat down to simmer. Cook until the egg starts to separate from the sides of the pan. (about 5 to 6 minutes). Heat your broiler and place the pan on the center rack and cook until brown, place back on stove with simmer heat and check the center with a knife. Eggs should be set and firm.

To serve cut the Fritata in 4 pieces pie shaped and serve on a 10 inch plate. Add some sliced tomatoes along the edge with a dribble of Balsamic vinegar on top and some salt and pepper.

Poached Eggs on Muffins

The famous name is Eggs Benedict but that's because of the benedict sauce used over the top of the eggs. Personally I have never liked the sauce so I would order it without. This is a variation of that recipe.

Prep Time: 5 minutes
Cook Time: 5 minutes
Servings: 2

2 whole wheat english muffins
4 eggs
4 slices deli ham, lean or lean canadian bacon
salt & pepper to taste

In a 2 or 3 quart saucepan heat water to a boil. When boiling shut off heat and add each egg separately (look below how to poach an egg) and cook for 3 to 4 minutes if you want soft centers and hard whites. Remove eggs with slotted spoon and let drain.

In a small non stick skillet fry the ham, while the eggs are cooking, until slightly brown around the edges.

Toast the english muffins, set on plate open faced and place 1 slice of the browned ham on each half of muffin, then place one egg on top of each piece of ham. Salt and pepper to taste.

On the side serve some cut fresh fruit cut up in a bowl.

How to poach an egg:
I had a lot of trouble at first. Maybe this will help you. Crack the egg into a shallow dish. Just before putting the egg in the water, stir the water to make it swirl. Slip the egg from the shallow dish into the middle of the swirl. Make sure to follow the motion of the swirl with the dish so the egg goes into the water in the same direction.

Blueberry Orange Oat Muffins

Great taste and good for you. How can you beat it? You can bake these and freeze them for a quick healthy breakfast or snack.

Prep time: 15 minutes
Cook Time: 15 minutes
Serving: 12

½ cup rolled oats
½ cup low fat buttermilk
1 ½ cups whole wheat flour
1 teaspoon baking powder
½ teaspoon baking soda
½ teaspoon ground cinnamon
¼ teaspoon salt
1 medium orange
½ cup Splenda sugar substitute
¼ cup canola oil
¼ cup egg substitute
1 cup blueberries, fresh is best but frozen will work

In a small bowl combine oats and buttermilk and set aside for 5 minutes.

Preheat oven to 400 degrees F. Lightly coat 12 muffin cups with cooking spray.

Whisk flour, baking powder, baking soda, cinnamon and salt together in a medium bowl.

Grate rind from the orange and add to a large bowl, squeeze ⅓ cup orange juice and add to rind. Whisk in sugar substitute, oil and egg until mixture is smooth. Blend in oatmeal mixture from 1st bowl, followed by flour mixture from second bowl. Stir until ingredients are just combined, then gently fold in berries.

Spoon batter into prepared muffin tins and bake for 15 minutes, or until a tooth pick inserted in center of muffin comes out clean. Let cool.

Apple Walnut Pancakes

Another version of whole wheat pancakes. I just love pancakes. Top with fresh fruit for a great breakfast.

Prep time: 15 minutes
Cook Time: 15 minutes
Servings: 8 pancakes

1 cup whole wheat flour
¼ cup oat flour (oats ground into flour consistency)
¼ cup chopped toasted pecans
1 ½ teaspoons brown sugar substitute from Sugar Twin
1 ½ teaspoons baking powder
¼ teaspoon salt
1 cup coarsely shredded & peeled granny smith apple
¾ cup skim milk
¼ cup apple juice
1 tablespoon canola oil
½ teaspoon vanilla extract
1 egg

In a large bowl stir in whole wheat flour, oat flour, pecans, brown sugar substitute, baking powder and salt. Stir till mixed, add apple, toss.

In a smaller bowl combine milt, oil, vanilla and egg, stir well. Then add to flour mixture, stirring till smooth.

On a hot nonstick griddle or skillet spoon about ⅓ cup batter for each pancake. Turn when tops are covered with bubbles and edges look cooked.

High protein Oat Waffles

Use a good-quality, non-stick waffle iron. A little tip: you can make the waffles ahead of time and freeze in an airtight container. Reheat in a toaster.

Makes 10 waffles (allow 2 or 3 per person)

Soaking time: Overnight
Preparation time: 5 minutes
Cooking time: 8 minutes per batch in your waffle maker

½ cup dried cannellini, white kidney or great northern beans
2¼ cups water
1¾ cups old-fashioned oats (or brown rice flakes)
2 small packages sweet & low or equal or 1 tablespoon agave nectar
¾ tablespoon whole flaxseed
1 tablespoon baking powder
1½ teaspoons vanilla extract
1 teaspoon salt
Fresh strawberries or blueberries for topping

The night before, place the beans in a large bowl and cover with water, refrigerate. In the morning, drain the beans discarding the soaking water. Place in a blender with 2¼ cups fresh water and the oats, nectar, flaxseed, baking powder, vanilla and salt. Blend until smooth, light and foamy. Set aside and preheat a non-stick waffle iron.

Pour 1/3 cup of batter onto the hot waffle iron for each 10-cm (4-inch) waffle, close the iron and cook for at least 8 minutes. If the iron is hard to open, let the waffle cook for another minute or two.

Repeat with the remaining batter, blending briefly before pouring each waffle. If the batter thickens while standing, add just enough water to return it to its original consistency. The waffles should be golden brown and crisp.

Serve immediately with fresh strawberries or blueberries.

Bran Muffins with Applesauce

Low fat, low sugar bran muffins everyone will enjoy.

Prep Time: 10 minutes
Cook Time: 20 minutes
Servings: 4, 12 small muffins

6 slices whole wheat bread, torn in small pieces
¾ ounce bran or oat bran cereal, low sugar
½ teaspoon baking soda
⅔ cup non fat dry milk
10 teaspoons of Splenda artificial sugar
1 ½ teaspoons honey
4 teaspoons olive oil
¾ cup egg substitute
1 banana sliced thin and cubed
1 cup unsweetened applesauce

Preheat the oven to 375 degrees. Spray a muffin pan with non stick cooking spray. Mix the whole wheat bread, bran, baking soda, non fat dry milk, splenda, honey, olive oil and egg substitute in a medium bowl.

Stir in the banana and applesauce lightly until just combined.

Bake for 15 to 20 minutes.

Caramel Apple Coffee Cake

Prep Time: 20 minutes
Cook Time: 40 minutes
Servings: 8

½ cup plus 2 Tablespoon unbleached flour
½ cup whole wheat pastry flour
¾ cup brown sugar twin, sugar substitute
½ teaspoon ground cinnamon
¾ teaspoon baking soda
¼ cup plus 2 Tablespoon nonfat or low-fat buttermilk
¼ cup egg substitute
1 tsp. vanilla extract
3 Granny Smith apples, diced into ⅓ inch pieces

Place the flours, brown sugar substitute and cinnamon in a medium sized bowl and stir to mix well, using the back of the spoon to press out any lumps in the brown sugar substitute. Add baking soda and stir to mix well. Add buttermilk, egg substitute, vanilla extract and apples to the flour mixture. Stir to mix well. The batter will be thick.

Coat a 9" round baking pan with nonstick spray and spread batter evenly in pan. Sprinkle the topping over the batter. (see topping below)

Bake at 325 for 35-40 minutes or just until top springs back when lightly touched. You can also use a clean wooden toothpick to insert in center and check for dryness. Be careful not to over-bake.

Let cool to room temp for at least 30 min and cut into wedges. Serve warm or at room temperature.

Topping:
1/4 cup whole wheat pastry flour
1/4 cup brown sugar substitute by Sugar Twin
1/3 cup honey crunch wheat germ or chopped toasted pecans
1 Tablespoon plus 1 tsp. unsweetened applejuice

To make topping place the flour, sugar and wheat germ or nuts into a small bowl, and mix well. Add juice concentrate and stir until mixture is moist and crumbly. Add more juice if needed.

Coffee Ring with Fresh Raspberry's

Prep Time: 15 minutes
Cook Time: 45 minutes
Servings: 12

1 cup unbleached flour
½ cup whole wheat flour
½ cup brown sugar substitute, Sugar Twin
⅔ cup oat bran
1 teaspoon baking soda
½ cup unsweetened apple sauce
1 ¼ cup vanilla low fat yogurt
½ teaspoon grated lemon rind (zest)
1 large egg lightly beaten
1 large egg white lightly beaten
1 cup raspberries
1 tablespoon all purpose flour
2 teaspoons skim milk

In a large bowl combine the flour, whole wheat flour, brown sugar substitute, oat bran and baking soda. Make a well in the center of the mixture. In a small bowl combine the applesauce, yogurt, lemon rind, egg and egg white. Combine with dry ingredients, stirring until just moist.

In a small bowl combine raspberries and 1 tablespoon flour, toss gently to coat. Fold raspberries into the batter.

Spoon batter into a 6 cup Bundt pan coated with cooking spray.

Bake at 350 degrees for 45 minutes or until wooden pick inserted in the center comes out clean. Let cool 10 minutes on wire rack, remove from pan. Let cool completely on rack.

Breakfast Milkshake

A milkshake for Breakfast? You may think it's silly, but this low fat, high fiber nutrition drink is so good your kids will gulp it down and I bet you will too.

Prep time: 3 minutes

8 ounces non fat yogurt either lemon or blueberry flavored
½ cup blueberries
1 teaspoon vanilla
Honey to taste

Combine in a blender and whirl until smooth

Pour into a 8 ounce glass and enjoy.

Breakfast Ham & Cheese Strata
(Crock Pot Recipe)

This is great for those days that you have plans in the morning, like going to church, and would love to have a brunch made when you return.

Prep Time: 20 minutes
Cook Time: 3 hours
Servings: 8

1 tablespoon Smart Balance
8 slices sourdough bread, remove crusts & break into small pieces
6 ounces thinly sliced ham, roughly chopped
8 ounces shredded low fat Monterey Jack cheese (reserve ½ cup)
½ small onion, minced, separated
1 ½ cups egg substitute
3 ¼ cups fat free half and half
½ teaspoon salt
½ teaspoon pepper
⅓ teaspoon hot sauce (like Tabasco)

Cut the bread into 16 triangles and toast in 250 degree oven for 3 to 4 minutes.

Grease the crock pot with the tablespoon of Smart Balance.

Place 8 of the bread triangles into the bottom of the crock pot, sprinkle in the small pieces of crusts so that the bottom of the crock pot is covered in bread. Add the ham, sprinkling it over the bread to make a layer. Add the cheese reserving the ½. Sprinkle 1 tablespoon of the onions over the cheese, top with the remaining 8 bread triangles and set aside.

In a large bowl combine the eggs, half and half, salt, pepper, and hot sauce, whisk until blended. Pour the egg mix over the bread, sprinkle with remaining onions. Let sit 15 minutes then sprinkle the remaining ½ cup of cheese over.

Cover and cook on low 3 hours. Remove the lid and let rest for 10 minutes before cutting and serving.

Lunch including Salads

Quick lunches in my house are the regular. Some of them are my personal favorites. I always keep some garlic and jalepeno wraps (tortillas) in the refrigerator. I top them with 2 slices of low fat lunch meat, *(maybe ham or turkey)* a slice of jarlsberg *(lite)* cheese, spicy brown mustard and lettuce. Roll it and enjoy it. I sometimes do the same with a whole wheat english muffin or even a sandwich with some fresh sliced 7 grain bread picked up at the bakery.

Another idea is to cut up a fruit bowl with whatever is fresh in the house, apples, mangoes, strawberry's, blueberries, grapes, or orange slices. Even great if you make it the night before, put it in a bowl and cover with plastic wrap and put it in the refrigerator.

Sometimes I like to just take a head of iceberg lettuce, cut in in half, put in on a plate and pour some fat free, low sugar dressing on top. I get a little more complicated at times, especially if I am in the mood for a real salad. Then my favorite is to take a handful or two of mixed greens, cut up some romaine lettuce, add a half of cucumber sliced, some cubes of roma tomatoes, throw in a couple slices of onion, then sprinkle some garlic powder, pepper, one tablespoon of extra virgin cold pressed olive oil and three or four tablespoons of balsamic vinegar. Sprinkle a bit of water on top, then toss it well. *(yum!)*

Like the breakfast recipes the following are for the special days and the weekends.

Cucumber Salad with Sesame Tabasco Dressing

Prep time: 15 minutes
Servings: 3 to 4

2 cucumbers peeled and sliced
½ bell pepper sliced julienne style
½ onion chopped coarse
3 tablespoon olive oil
1 tablespoon lemon juice
1 tablespoon lime juice
2 gloves garlic crushed
15 drops tabasco sauce
2 tablespoons sesame seeds
2 tablespoons white wine vinegar

In a large bowl combine everything and mix well. Serve in separate smaller bowls.

Tuna Melt

Prep Time: 20 minutes
Cook Time: 10 minutes
Servings: 4

2 cans water packed tuna
4 english muffins split and toasted
⅓ cup celery, chopped fine
¼ cup green onions or regular yellow onions chopped
2 tablespoons light mayonnaise
1 egg white (optional) cooked
1 teaspoon prepared mustard
4 slices reduced fat swiss cheese
1 tomato sliced
4 leaves romaine or iceberg lettuce (optional)

Drain tuna and place in bowl flaking it with fork to separate. Add celery, onions, mayonnaise, cooked egg white and mustard. Mix well.

Preheat oven to 350 degrees. Form or spoon tuna mixture onto muffins placed on oven proof dish or foil. Bake for 10 to 15 minutes, remove, add slice of cheese on top and bake for 2 or 3 minutes or more to melt cheese.
Serve with tomato slice on top and lettuce on the side.

Palm Heart Salad

Prep time: 30 min
Servings: 4 to 6

For the dressing:
½ lime or lemon, juiced
1 teaspoon whole-grain mustard
1 tablespoon white wine vinegar
½ package sugar substitute or 1 teaspoon Splenda
¼ cup extra-virgin olive oil
Salt and freshly ground black pepper
To make the dressing: Mix the first 4 ingredients and then drizzle olive oil in slowly while stirring constantly. Season with salt and pepper, to taste.

For the salad:
1 (14 or 15-ounce) can palm hearts, drained and sliced crosswise
2 ripe mangoes, peeled and thinly sliced
2 ripe avocados (or 1 large), peeled, stoned, and thinly sliced
½ cucumber, peeled and thinly sliced
½ Scotch bonnet (or other hot chile pepper,) de-seeded and finely chopped
½ lime or lemon (to be squeezed on the avocado to prevent discoloring)

Assemble all the salad ingredients in a bowl and serve the dressing on the side.

Asparagus & Pinenut Salad

A super easy vegetable side dish to complement any meal.
This recipe is better when the dressing is prepared in advance.

Prep Time: 5 minutes
Cooking Time: 5 minutes
Ready in: 10 minutes
Servings: 4

2 bunches asparagus
2 tbsp pinenuts
1 lemon
2 tbsp olive oil
2 tsp fresh rosemary
Pinch of black pepper

Wash the lemon to remove any waxy coating. Zest (look below) the skin of the lemon avoiding any white pith. Juice half the remaining lemon. Combine the zest, lemon juice, olive oil and rosemary together and set aside.
Trim the asparagus spears, snapping the woody end off with your hand. Wash and steam for 3 minutes. Plunge the spears into cold water to stop further cooking.
Dry roast the pine nuts in a small pan until slightly golden.

To serve drizzle the dressing over the cooked asparagus. Top with pine nuts and season with black pepper.

Zesting: is the art of removing little shards of skin without going into the fruit. You can buy a zesting tool at your local restaurant supply.

Asian Salad

There is no hard and fast rule about which greens you choose, but it's nice if you are making an Asian salad to select leaves with an exotic air to them. I use a mixture you can buy at most grocery stores called Spring Mix.

Prep Time:10 minutes
Ready in:20 minutes
Servings: 4 to 6

4 handfuls of Mixed greens
1 cup snow peas
1/3 cup olive oil
1 tbsp marin (this is a low alcohol rice wine)
1 tbsp brown rice vinegar
½ tbsp tamari (tamari is soy sauce made without wheat) or lite soy sauce.
1 clove garlic crushed

Wash and dry the salad greens in a salad spinner. String the snow peas and arrange all the greens on a platter.

 To make the dressing, mix the ingredients in a jar or bowl. Pour over the greens and serve immediately.

You can make up the dressing in advance and keep it in a jar in the fridge.

Salad with Carrot Ginger Dressing

Prep Time: 10 minutes
Servings Salad: 2 to 4
Servings Dressing: 8 so refrigerate remaining and use later.

In your favorite Salad mixing bowl put 4 large handfuls of mixed greens (your choice) I like to add a half of a cucumber, some green pepper, ½ onion sliced and maybe some broccoli or yellow squash.

Dressing:
1/2 pound carrots (3 medium), chopped
1/4 cup water
1/4 cup seasoned rice vinegar
3 tablespoons minced peeled fresh ginger
1 tablespoon soy sauce
1 tablespoon Asian sesame oil
1 shallot, chopped
1 tablespoon sherry
½ cup peanut oil.

In a blender, combine the carrot, water, vinegar, ginger, soy sauce, sesame oil, shallot and sherry and puree. While the motor is running, drizzle in the oil until incorporated. Store in the refrigerator until ready to use.

Mango & Avocado Salad with Grilled Chicken

Prep time: 45 minutes
Cook Time: 15 minutes
Servings: 4

2 whole skinned chicken breasts cut in half either sliced about 3/8 inch thick or pounded.
2 limes juiced
½ teaspoon salt
1 teaspoon ground cumin
2 small or 1 large avocados, peeled and cut into 2 inch dice.
2 medium size mangoes, peeled and cut into 2 inch dice.
2 cucumbers, seeded and cut into thin half moons
4 tablespoons olive oil
2 cups cilantro leaves, washed
1 scallion trimmed
2 tablespoons white wine vinegar
Fresh ground black pepper

Trim the chicken of fat. combine half the lime juice with the ground cumin and a pinch of salt, rub over the chicken. Grill the chicken on the Bar-b or in a grill pan for about 6 minutes each side. Remove to a cutting board. Let cool a bit and cut the chicken on a diagonal into thin slices, set aside.

In a blender or food processor, puree the olive oil cilantro, scallion with the white wine vinegar and a little salt and pepper.

Combine in a bowl the avocados, mangoes, cucumbers and remaining lime juice. Season with a pinch of salt and some ground pepper to taste. Divide and arrange the mango/ avocado mixture on 4 dinner plates. Arrange the grilled sliced chicken over the mango & avocado then spoon the dressing over the chicken.

Spicy Peanut Angel Hair Salad

Prep Time: 15 minutes
Cooking Time: 8 minutes
Servings: 4

1 pound Angel hair Pasta
⅔ cup creamy peanut butter from a health food store. Oil drained.
1 tablespoon sesame oil
⅓ cup rice or red wine vinegar
1 teaspoon red chile flakes
2 small packages sweet & Low or Equal
1 tablespoon Dijon mustard
1 tablespoon coarse ground coriander
2 tablespoons soy sauce (lite)
⅓ cup canola or olive oil
1 cucumber, sliced in half and then in slices
1 red bell pepper, julienne
1 bunch scallions, sliced
1/2 cup chopped roasted (salted) peanuts for garnish (not necessary)

Cook the spaghetti, al dante, drain and set aside.

In a small bowl, whisk together the peanut butter, sesame oil, vinegar, chile, artificial sweetener, Dijon, coriander and soy until smooth. Whisk in the canola or olive oil.

In a large bowl, toss dressing with the pasta, cucumbers, bell pepper and scallions. Taste and add ground pepper if necessary.

Separate into 4 servings on a dinner plate and garnish with peanuts.

Vegetable Casserole with Goat Cheese

You can make this delicious casserole the night before or when you have time. Either refrigerate or even freeze, heat and serve.

Prep Time: 20 minutes
Cook Time: 55 minutes
Servings: 6

4 tablespoons olive oil
1 medium onion sliced ½ inch
1 medium red bell pepper slice ½ inch
⅓ cup garlic chopped (about 16 cloves)
½ eggplant, peeled, sliced thin
7 roma tomatoes sliced thin
2 large zucchini sliced thin
3 tablespoons chopped fresh thyme, oregano and parsley
8 oz soft mild goat cheese

Heat 2 tablespoons olive oil in skillet and saute onion and pepper slices about 5 minutes. Add ½ the garlic and cook 1 minute. Spread this on the bottom of a 9 x 13 inch glass baking dish.

Arrange eggplant evenly over pepper and onion, season with salt and pepper, then top with alternate rows of tomato, zucchini, overlapping slightly. Season with more salt & pepper. Sprinkle with the herbs and remaining garlic. Drizzle remaining 2 tablespoons olive oil over top. Bake in preheated 350 degree F oven until tender, about 50 minutes. Baste occasionally with pan juices.

Sprinkle crumbled goat cheese over the top, bake 5 min until cheese melts.

Try serving it over a slice of toasted Whole Wheat bread. Enjoy

Crab on Muffins

This is a quick lunch your friends will really be impressed with. (so will hubby)

Prep Time: 15 minutes
Cook Time; 15 minutes
Servings: 2

2 whole wheat english muffins fork split in half and toasted
1 cup imitation crabmeat, chopped coarse
¼ cup onion, chopped
⅛ cup green pepper, chopped
1 plum tomato chopped
¼ cup pitted black olives, chopped
2 pitted black olives, sliced in half
½ cup low fat sour cream
¾ teaspoon dill
½ cup grated course swiss or monterey jack cheese
Shake of paprika

In a large bowl mix crab meat, onion, pepper, tomato, chopped olives, sour cream and dill. Stir well.

Place the toasted english muffin on a tin foiled cookie sheet, place ½ cup of the above mixture on top of each ½ of muffin. Bake for 15 minutes, sprinkle shredded cheese on top, turn on broiler and watch closely till cheese melts and turns brown. Remove, place 2 half's on each plate.

Garnish with one half olive on each half, sprinkle with paprika.

Vegetable Lasagna

This dish is one of my favorite. If you have any left over freeze it in either plastic wrap or a zip lock in individual portions. Heat in micro when you need a quick lunch. You won't believe how good this is and without meat.

Prep Time: 20 min
Cook Time: Micro 20 minutes
Cook Time: Oven 1 hr 10 min
Servings: 8

1 15 oz container nonfat ricotta cheese
1 10 oz package frozen chopped spinach, thawed and drained
½ cup egg substitute
⅓ cup parmesan cheese, grated
¼ cup parsley, chopped
¼ teaspoon ground nutmeg
¼ teaspoon crushed red pepper flakes
3 ½ cups prepared tomato sauce
9 lasagna noodles, uncooked
¼ cup red lentils, uncooked
1 ½ cups shredded nonfat mozzarella cheese (6 oz)

In a large bowl combine ricotta cheese, spinach, egg, 2 tablespoon parmesan cheese, parsley, nutmeg and red pepper. Mix until blended.

Pour 1 cup of the tomato sauce into an 11x 7 inch glass baking dish. Spread over bottom. Arrange 3 noodles in layer on top of sauce. Spoon ⅓ rd of ricotta mixture over noodles. Sprinkle 2 tablespoons lentils, ½ cup mozzarella and remaining parmesan over the top. Pour 1 ½ cups tomato sauce over cheese. Arrange another layer of noodles, repeat layering using remaining ingredients. Top layer should be noodles, then ricotta mixture and topped with mozzarella.

Preheat the oven to 350 degrees F, Cover with tin foil tight and bake for 1 hour, remove foil and bake 10 minutes.

Let stand 10 minutes before serving.

GRILLED CHICKEN, QUESADILLA

What a lunch or dinner! I just love Quesadilla's. Your family will love them also.

Prep time: 15 minutes
Cook time: 15 minutes
Servings: 4

2 large boneless chicken breasts
Olive oil
Salt and freshly ground pepper
2 small or 1 large onion chopped course
1 green pepper sliced
4 - 9 inch spinach or Jalapeno tortillas
1 cup Monterey Jack (low fat) cheese, grated
1 cup Cheddar cheese (low fat) , grated
4 heads of garlic chopped
2 tablespoons finely chopped fresh thyme
Salt and freshly ground pepper

Preheat grill or large pan. Brush chicken with olive oil and season with salt and pepper to taste. Grill for 5 minutes on each side or until cooked through, remove and let rest. Toss peppers and onions with the garlic and thyme in 1 tablespoon olive oil (same pan) and season with salt and pepper to taste. Cook until onions are translucent.

Place ½ the tortillas on a flat surface. Divide both cheeses among the tortillas. Slice chicken on the bias into 1/4-inch thick slices. Place on tortillas and layer the onions and peppers on top. Top the four tortillas with the remaining four tortillas. Brush the top with olive oil and season with salt and pepper to taste. Grill, oil side down until golden brown. Carefully flip over and continue grilling until golden brown and the cheese has melted.

Avocado with Crab

My wife Mardy makes this quite often. Wow ! is it good. Very low in fat with a taste you won't believe.

Prep Time: 10 minutes
Cook Time: 5 minutes
Serves: 2

1 Avocado, sliced in half, pit removed
1 cup imitation crab meat
⅓ cup non fat sour cream
1 plum tomato, chopped
¼ cup onion, chopped
¼ cup green pepper, chopped
¼ cup swiss cheese, grated coarse
Salt & pepper to taste
⅛ teaspoon Dill

In a bowl combine the imitation crab meat, sour cream, tomato, onion, green pepper, and dill. Add salt and pepper to taste.

Lay the avocado on a dish that can be microwaved and put in the oven. I use a small stoneware dish that fits one half the avocado and serve in the same dish. Spoon the crab meat mixture over the top of the avocado filling the void from the pit and just letting it spill over the sides.

Place in microwave on high for one minute to warm. Sprinkle ½ the cheese over each avocado. Place under broiler for 3 minutes to melt the cheese into the crab mixture.

Serve

Dinners

Let's take a minute and talk about dinners. When I was growing up my mother use to place the pans on the table and everyone would serve themselves. When ever company came over she would set the table with silverware, linen tablecloth, nice linen napkins (*usually hand crocheted*) and would present her meals in large serving bowls and platters. My Italian mothers meals were, I know now, very high calorie, carb loaded, full fat foods. Mom had no idea, nor concern about fat, sugar, carbohydrates or cholesterol. For her, food and it's preparation was a true expression of her love. I adored her meals and her recipes, and still do today. Knowing better now, I have revised these favorites into low fat/ low sugar/ low cholesterol renditions. Do these precious recipes taste the same? Close...., acceptable to be sure, but not exactly the same. Perhaps if she were still here to stir the pot............

Why am I telling you this? Because you need to take all those old favorites and either put them aside or change them so the fat and sugar content is lower. How do we do this? For the fat part we can use low fat ingredients, for example: skim milk or 1% milk instead of whole milk. No fat half and half, no fat coffee creamer, low fat cheese etc. Use olive or canola oil instead of vegetable oil. Smart Balance or Cant Believe it's Not Butter instead of margarine or real butter. For white sugar we can use either Splenda or a sugar substitute like Equal or Sweet and Low, and for brown sugar we can use Sugar Twin brown sugar substitute. For meats you can change what you buy. Ground meat is now marked with percentages of fat, (try to stay under 10%.) Buy lean cuts of beef. Try and stay away or limit pork. With chicken, always take the skin off, as with any fowl. Buy turkey sausage and turkey cuts of lunch meat.

You would be surprised just by using the above 'little hints' how much you will reduce the amount of fat and sugar you would have ingesting.

Secondly, I would like to see you switch to preparing the plate for each person in the kitchen, like a restaurant does, and not serve family style with the bowls or pans on the table. You would be amazed at how much less you will eat. (*no seconds, remember*)

With each of the following dinners pick a side dish from the next category. Some of the dinners are so complete they do not require anything with them except for perhaps a salad.

Barbecue Chicken with Coffee Sauce

You won't believe the great taste of this one. When you first read it you can't visualize the coffee barbecue sauce. Once you taste it, you're hooked. Goes well with Fish also.

Prep time: 15 minutes
Cook time: 45 minutes
Ready in: 1 hour
Servings: 4

Ingredients:
1 whole chicken cut in pieces for barbecuing
¼ cup Worcestershire sauce
½ cup very strong coffee, espresso preferred
½ cup ketchup
½ cup red wine vinegar
3 fresh hot chili peppers or Jalapenos chopped
¼ cup dark brown sugar substitute by Sugar Twin
2 tablespoons hot dry mustard mixed with 1 tablespoon water
1 onion chopped fine
2 tablespoons cumin
2 cloves garlic, crushed
2 tablespoons chili powder
1 tablespoon dark molasses

Just combine all the ingredients, except the chicken, in a saucepan and simmer for 20 minutes, cool, then puree in blender, strain.

When the chicken has cooked on the barbecue for about 30 minutes turn the flame down to low and start basting for the remaining 10 to 15 minutes.

Chicken Rollatini

This is chicken smothered in parmesan cheese and rolled with mozzarella and prosciutto and baked in white wine."

Prep Time:15 Minutes
Cook Time:30 Minutes
Ready In:45 Minutes
Servings:4

INGREDIENTS:
4 skinless, boneless chicken breast halves
1/2 cup shredded Parmesan cheese
1 clove garlic, finely chopped
4 teaspoons smart balance
4 ounces thinly sliced prosciutto, no fat
10 ounces sliced skim milk mozzarella cheese
1/3 cup white wine
1/4 cup olive oil
1 pinch black pepper

DIRECTIONS:
Preheat oven to 325 degrees F (165 degrees C).

Pound chicken breasts flat, and lay them on work surface. Sprinkle liberally with Parmesan cheese on both sides. Place a pinch of minced garlic and 1 teaspoon smart balance in the center of each breast. Cover each breast with a layer of prosciutto and mozzarella cheese. Reserve some of the prosciutto to place on top of the chicken. Roll up each chicken breast, and secure with toothpicks.

In a 9x13 inch baking dish, combine white wine and olive oil. Arrange chicken rolls in dish. Place a small piece of prosciutto on top of each roll, and sprinkle with pepper.

Bake in preheated oven for 30 minutes, or until chicken is no longer pink, an juices run clear.

Thai Red Chicken Curry

A quick and easy curry stir-fry made with chicken, zucchini, red bell pepper and carrot. Coconut milk and curry paste make an irresistible sauce. No need to go out to eat, as this dish is ready in about 20 minutes!

Prep Time: 10 Min
Cook Time: 10 Min
Ready in: 20 Min
Servings: 4

INGREDIENTS
2 teaspoons olive oil
1 pound skinless, boneless chicken breast halves - cut into thin strips
1 tablespoon Thai red curry paste
1 cup sliced halved zucchini
1 red bell pepper, seeded and sliced into strips
1/2 cup sliced carrots
1 onion, quartered then halved
1 tablespoon cornstarch or flour for thickening.
1 (14 ounce) can light coconut milk
2 tablespoons chopped fresh cilantro

Heat the oil in a large skillet over medium-high heat. Add the chicken pieces; cook and stir for about 3 minutes. Mix in the curry paste, zucchini, bell pepper, carrot and onion. Cook and stir for a few minutes.

Dissolve the cornstarch in the coconut milk, then pour into the skillet. Bring to a boil, then simmer over medium heat for 1 minutes. Right before serving, stir in the cilantro.

BOURBON-LACED CHICKEN WITH PEACHES

This baked chicken dish is low cal and delicious. You will have it on the table in less then an hour.

Prep time: 15 minutes
Cook Time: 45 minutes

2 whole chicken breasts split in half, bone in
½ teaspoon salt
1/8 teaspoon freshly ground black pepper
2 tablespoons smart balance spread
1 large onion, finely chopped
1 teaspoon paprika
1 ½ cups green onions, chopped
½ cup orange juice
2 tablespoons bourbon
1 cup chopped fresh peaches (about 2 medium peaches)
Dash nutmeg

Preheat oven to 400 degrees.
Sprinkle chicken breasts with salt and pepper. Place in a 13 by 9-inch baking pan and set aside.

In a medium skillet, melt the smart balance over medium heat. Add the chopped onion and cook, stirring occasionally, until translucent, about 5 minutes. Add the paprika and all but 1 tablespoon of the green onions and continue to cook, stirring occasionally, for an additional 4 minutes.

Spread the onion mixture evenly over the chicken, spoon the orange juice and bourbon over the top, and bake in the preheated oven for 30 minutes, turning and basting occasionally.

Remove the chicken from the oven, spoon the peaches over the top, sprinkle with nutmeg, and return to the oven for an additional 15 to 20 minutes or until the chicken is tender and shows no trace of pink near the bone. Remove the chicken from the pan, place on serving dish, and pour the juices over the chicken. Garnish with the remaining green onions and serve immediately

JAMAICAN JERKED CHICKEN

You have all heard of Jamaican Jerked Chicken. The great recipes of this dish are usually passed on family to family but never shared. This one is very special. The preparation may take a while, but is well worth it. When you serve it to your family or guests I guarantee everyone will be singing your praises. Let's get to it.

Prep time: 40 minutes
Cooking time: 50 minutes
Ready in: 1.5 hours
Marinade time: 24 hours. Make the sauce one day and cook it the next.
Servings: 8

2 whole chickens cut in pieces
2 cups distilled white vinegar, plus 1 teaspoon
2 cups finely chopped scallions
2 Scotch bonnets, seeded and minced (you can use habanero chili's)
2 tablespoons soy sauce
4 tablespoons fresh lime juice
5 teaspoons ground allspice
2 bay leaves
6 cloves garlic, minced
1 tablespoon salt
1 package sugar substitute
1 1/2 teaspoons dried thyme, crumbled
1 teaspoon cinnamon

In a large bowl pour the vinegar (reserve the 1 teaspoon) over the chicken, soak the chicken pieces turning them for 5 or 10 minutes, drain, transfer to 2 sealable plastic bags and set aside.

In the bowl of a food processor combine remaining 1 teaspoon vinegar, scallions, Scotch bonnets, soy sauce, lime juice, allspice, bay leaves, garlic, salt, sugar substitute, thyme, and cinnamon, process well to blend. Reserve 2 tablespoons of the jerk marinade for the Jamaican Barbecue Sauce.

Rinse the chicken pieces again well under cold running water and pat dry with paper towels. Divide chicken pieces between 2 heavy-duty gallon plastic sealable bags and divide marinade evenly between the two. Turn bags over to evenly distribute marinade, and refrigerate chicken for at least 24 hours and up to 2 days.

On an oiled grill rack set about 6 inches above red-hot coals, grill chicken (in batches if necessary), covered, for 15 to 20 minutes on each side, (total time 30 to 40 minutes) or until cooked through. Transfer to a warm platter and keep warm until serving.

Serve with Jamaican Barbecue Sauce, alongside baked plantains or wild rice.

Jamaican Barbecue Sauce:
1 1/4 cups ketchup
1/3 cup soy sauce
2 tablespoons Jamaican hot pepper sauce
2 tablespoons Jerk marinade (reserved from marinade recipe above)
3 scallions, minced
3 cloves garlic, minced
3 tablespoons minced fresh ginger
1/4 cup dark brown sugar substitute from Sugar Twin
1/3 cup distilled white vinegar
3 tablespoons dark rum

In a medium non stick saucepan combine all ingredients except rum and bring to a boil, stirring to dissolve sugar. Reduce heat to a simmer and continue to cook another 12 minutes, until sauce is thick and flavorful and coats the back of a spoon.

Remove from heat and stir in rum. Cool sauce to room temperature before serving.

Chicken With Prunes

This is a great dish although it takes a bit of time to prepare. Do not get discouraged as the results will be worth it.

Prep Time: 20 minutes
Cook Time: 1 hours 30 minutes
Servings: 4

1/5 cup olive oil
1 (2-ounce) slice speck, finely chopped (Speck is a smoked raw ham that has an intense dry cured flavor. Use a smoked ham as a substitute.
1 chicken, cut into 8 pieces rinsed and dried
Salt and pepper
2 leeks thinly sliced use only the white part
12 shallots, finely chopped
2 teaspoons fresh thyme, minced
1 bay leaf
2 cups dry white wine
1 cup chicken broth
12 dried prunes, soaked for 1 hour in ½ -cup warm brandy

Warm the olive oil in a large, heavy casserole and cook the speck (ham) until light golden brown. Remove it to a plate, using a slotted spoon.

Season the chicken with salt and pepper and brown it on both sides in the same pan, then remove it to a plate. Add the leeks and shallots and saute. Add the thyme, bay leaf, wine, and chicken stock, scraping the bottom of the pot with a wooden spoon to dislodge the browned bits. Bring to a simmer and return the chicken to the casserole.

Cover the casserole loosely and simmer for 30 minutes. Add the soaked prunes and their liquids and simmer another 30 minutes, until the chicken is very tender and falling off the bone.

Remove the chicken to a plate and add the sauteed speck (ham) to the pan. Reduce the sauce for 5 minutes and season with salt and pepper. Return the chicken and to the sauce, shut the heat off and let rest to cool, then reheat gently and serve.

Grilled or Barbecued Chicken with Mango & Pineapple

Please don't make this in the first month. After that serve it on a special occasion. A tropical delight. Very simple and delicious. You can grill the chicken in a pan or place it on the Barbecue. Either way, you will get praises. Great with fresh asparagus.

Prep time: 15 minutes
Cooking time: 20 minutes

Canola or olive oil to cook with.
4 ½ chicken breasts
1 red onion, 1/4-inch slices
1 medium carrot, 1/4-inch bias slices
4 cloves of garlic, 1/16-inch slices
1 tablespoon minced ginger
2 serrano chile's, minced or some other hot chile's minced.
1 small pineapple, 1/2-inch dice
1 large mango, 1/2-inch dice
2 oranges, zested and juiced
1 lemon, zested and juiced
Salt and black pepper, to taste

Make the sauce in a large saucepan coated lightly with oil on medium heat, saute the onions, carrot, garlic, ginger and chile's. Stir and season with salt and pepper. Cook until soft, about 5 minutes. Add the pineapple, mango and citrus juices/zest. Bring to a boil and simmer for a 20 percent reduction, about 15 minutes. Set aside.

In a grill pan or on a bar-b grill the chicken breasts until done about 10 to fifteen minutes.

Place the chicken on a plate and cover with the sauce.

Spinach Lasagna...without the Noodles

Wait till you try this one, no noodles but great all the same.

1 pound ground beef
3 (14 oz)cans of sliced stewed tomatoes, drained
1 package of frozen chopped spinach, thawed, drained and heated
24 oz cottage cheese, (I use small curds)
2 cups of shredded mozzarella cheese
1/4 cup parmesan cheese
1 tablespoons oregano
2 tablespoons basil, dried but fresh would be better!
2 teaspoon garlic powder or more to taste
½ teaspoon pepper to taste.

Thaw and heat spinach in microwave until hot

Brown beef and add 2 cans of tomatoes and 1/2 carton of cottage cheese, add spices and simmer down until liquid is almost gone...will be a reddish color and the cottage cheese will liquify.

Put thawed/hot spinach in casserole 9x13 dish, add the meat mixture over the spinach then ½ the mozzarella cheese and add the last can of tomatoes, sprinkle some parmesan cheese.

Cover with shredded cheese.

Bake at 400 degrees for 15 minutes until bubbly and then broil for a few minutes until top browns a bit.

Baked Grouper or Cod with Ginger

You can bring this one in under ½ hour.. Other species of fish that work well with this dish include kingfish, snapper or even salmon. To ensure the fish is cooked evenly, select pieces of consistent thickness end to end.

Prep Time: 10 minutes
Cooking Time: 20 minutes
Ready in: 30 minutes

Servings: 1

1/2 pound mushrooms, try to use a mixture of different mushrooms like brown, shitake, oyster etc.
1 fillet of Fish, size is up to you and how hungry you are.
1 clove garlic , crushed
1 piece fresh ginger grated or 2 tablespoons of powdered ginger
1 tbsp tamari of lite soy sauce
1 tsp sesame oil
2 small bunches bok choy washed and leaves trimmed

Preheat oven to 350 degrees Make a parcel with a piece of double thickness foil. Wipe the mushrooms of dirt and cut into slices. Smear each side of the fish fillet with half the amount of grated ginger. In a small bowl mix the mushrooms with the remaining ginger, garlic, sesame oil and tamari (soy sauce) . Lay the mushrooms onto the foil. Wrap the foil parcel securely leaving space above the mushrooms to add the fish (later). Place in the oven and cook for 15 minutes.

While the mushrooms are cooking, wash and trim the bok choy, and set aside.

With 4 minutes cooking time remaining, heat a non stick frying pan with the sesame oil. Sear each side of the fish for 1 minute each side and season with black pepper. Remove the mushrooms from the oven and carefully open the parcel. Drop the fish onto the top of the mushrooms, secure the parcel again and return to the oven for a further 4 minutes.

Using the same pan cook the bok choy in the remaining sesame oil for 3 minutes until cooked. Remove the fish and mushrooms from the oven and serve with accompanying bok choy.

CRABMEAT CREPE

For this recipe you can used bought crepes or you can make them from scratch with the recipe below. Personally, I like to make the crepes. They're simple to make and everyone is impressed at your cooking abilities.

Prep Time: 15 min
Cook Time: 15 min
Servings: 2

1 cup Imitation crabmeat cut in 1" lengths and placed in bowl.
1 cup mushrooms chopped
1/2 cup sliced green onion
3 tablespoon smart balance
½ cup white wine (your choice)
Pinch salt
grind pepper
½ teaspoon   tarragon
1 can evaporated skim milk
2 to 3 Tablespoons Flour

Melt the margarine in large skillet, saute green onion and mushrooms, add salt and pepper to taste. The mushrooms will start to release a liquid. When they do add the white wine.
Sprinkle in the flour stirring well. Slowly add evaporated milk stirring until the mixture reaches the desired thickness. (you won't need the entire can) Add tarragon. Remove from heat.
Place the crabmeat in a bowl and pour enough sauce to cover the crabmeat, mixing well. Reserve the remaining cream sauce.

Divide the crabmeat mixture among your 4 or 5 crepes. Place some stuffing down the center of the crepe then fold the right and left side over.

In the large skillet put a tablespoon or so of olive oil with very low heat. Put the finished crepes in the skillet and cover. Turn frequently until heated thoroughly. (light brown)

Reheat your leftover mushroom sauce in another pan, thinning if necessary with white wine. Place heated crepes on individual plates and pour some mushroom sauce over.

CREPES

Prep time: 10 minutes
Cook time: 2 minutes each

2	eggs
¾	cup milk skimmed milk
Pinch	salt
½	cup all purpose flour
1	tablespoon olive oil
	smart balance

Take the above ingredients and blend them in a blender or just whisk them in the bowl you are using until smooth, real smooth.

In a small (depending on the size of the crepes you want) frying pan (teflon or non stick) melt a little smart balance (half a spoon) with medium heat. When melted spoon in about 3 to 4 tablespoons of the above mixture until it covers the bottom of the pan very thin. Tilt the pan back and forth quickly to spread the mixture evenly. Cook for about one minute and check the bottom for a little brownness. The best spatula to use is one about 1 ½ inches wide by about 10 inches long. Turn over and cook the same amount of time on the other side.

Put a piece of saran or plastic wrap over a plate and place your finished crepes on the plastic rap. This way you can heat them later, just before using them.

Voila, you are a French Crepe maker. (*impressive, HUH ?*)

Baked Salmon or Steelhead Trout with Mint

Perfect for a nice large salmon or steelhead trout filet or two. Baked in the oven, and served with new potatoes sprinkled with chopped mint and a drizzle of olive oil, a crisp green salad with sliced avocado along side, you have a healthy and easy, yet elegant meal.

4 pounds, cleaned and fillet of Salmon or Steelhead trout.
1 cup white wine
¼ cup chervil or parsley, chopped
¼ cup fresh mint , chopped
¼ cup fresh dill chopped
¼ cup chives chopped
1 lime juiced
2 tbsp olive oil

Prep Time: 15 minutes
Cooking Time: 25 minutes
Ready in: 45 minutes
Servings: 4 to 6

Preheat the oven to 350 degrees.

Lay the fish on a large sheet of baking foil with plenty of foil around the outside to wrap it up in a tight parcel. Mix the wine, fresh herbs, olive oil and lime juice and pour it over the fish. Secure the foil around the fish and bake for 1 hour. Set aside to rest in the foil for a further 10 minutes before serving.

Stuffed Orange Roughy

Prep Time: 15 minutes
Cook Time: 35 minutes
Servings: 2

2 large orange roughy fillets
1 cup imitation crabmeat, chopped corse
¼ cup onion, chopped
⅛ cup green pepper, chopped
1 plum tomato chopped
½ cup low fat sour cream
¾ teaspoon dill
½ cup grated course swiss or monterey jack cheese
¼ cup italian bread crumbs
1 tablespoon italian bread crumbs
1 tablespoon smart balance
Shake of paprika

Wash & pat dry the 2 orange roughy fillets, place 1 fillet in oven proof dish sprayed lightly with cooking spray.

In a large bowl mix crab meat, onion, pepper, tomato, sour cream and dill and bread crumbs. Stir well.

Mold filling on top of fillet pressing filling tightly together. Lay second fillet on top of filling. Lightly spread smart balance on top. Sprinkle with 1 tablespoon bread crumbs. Lightly sprinkle paprika and dill over top.

Preheat oven to 350 degrees and bake for 30 minutes.

Serve on platter and cut to serve with metal spatula at the table.

Baked Whole Snapper

You can use a whole snapper or snapper filets. Try the whole snapper. Be sure you buy it cleaned and descaled.

Ingredients:

1½ kg (3 pounds) whole snapper cleaned
2 tbsp slivered almonds
1 cup fresh parsley finely chopped
1 tbsp lemon zest (see zesting on page 87) and the juice of 1 large lemon
1/3 cup olive oil

1 large clove garlic cut into fine slivers

Prep Time: 15 minutes
Cooking Time: 35 minutes
Ready in: 50 minutes

Preheat the oven to 350 degrees

In a dry pan, roast the almonds over a medium heat until they give off a delicious toasty aroma.

Mix the parsley with the lemon zest and lemon juice, then slowly pour in the olive oil while stirring to make a paste.

Score the outside of the fish about 1 cm deep a few times and stab garlic into the gashes. Smear the paste all over the inside and outside of the fish, pressing the mixture firmly into the cavity of the fish. Wrap the fish in foil and bake for 20 minutes. Remove the foil and bake for a further 10 - 15 minutes until the skin is crunchy

Asian Oven Baked Grouper of Flounder

Actually you can substitute a variety of fish including Snapper or Talipia. You will love the Asian taste.

Prep Time: 25 minutes
Marinade Time: 30 minutes
Cook Time: 30 minutes
Servings: 4

4 flounder fillets
2 tablespoons sake
2 tablespoons soy sauce
2 tablespoons fresh lime juice
2 teaspoons minced fresh ginger
2 teaspoons sesame oil
1 teaspoon honey
1 teaspoon lightly toasted sesame seeds
6 ounces shitake mushrooms, stemmed and thinly sliced
4 green onions, green tops only, cut into 1-inch pieces
1 large carrot, peeled and cut into 2-inch long matchstick strips
1/2 large red pepper, seeded and cut into thin strips
Smart balance

Lay the fish flat in a baking dish. In a bowl, whisk together the sake, soy sauce, lime juice, ginger, sesame oil, honey, and sesame seeds. Pour over the fish and let marinate for up to 30 minutes.

Preheat the oven to 375 degrees F. Cut 4 large squares of heavy aluminum foil large enough to hold 1 flounder fillet and one-quarter of the vegetables. Lightly smear some smart balance on 1 side of each filet and Arrange 1 fish fillet on each sheet of aluminum foil and top with one-quarter of the mushrooms, onions, carrots, peppers, and marinade. Wrap tightly and place on a baking sheet. Bake until the fish is cooked through and the vegetables are tender, 15 to 20 minutes. Remove from the oven and unwrap each package. Transfer the fish and vegetables to 4 large plates and top with the cooking juices.

Serve with Sauteed Shiitakes and hot wild rice.

PASTA with ROASTED VEGGIES AND CHICKEN

Prep Time: 15 minutes
Cooking time: 30 minutes

1 pound of your favorite pasta, I use linguine or spaghetti Plus (whole grain) from Barilla.

6	garlic cloves minced
1	red , green and yellow pepper sliced
1	green zucchini, quartered & sliced
1	onions , quartered and sliced
1	carrots into matchsticks

4 to 6 plum tomatoes quartered
1 to 2 Tbls olive oil
pinch salt
pepper ground to taste
½ teaspoon   basil
½ teaspoon marjoram
½ teaspoon rosemary
2 cups chicken broth thickened with a little corn starch

Lay all vegetables in non stick roasting pan, season w/salt, pepper, rosemary, basil, add olive oil and mix well till all vegetables are coated. Broil, stirring frequently till vegetables become crisp and browned, about 25 minutes.

Cook pasta, drain, season with salt & pepper, add roasted vegetables, stir well, add enough thickened chicken broth to coat pasta and vegetables.

Serve with parmesan cheese, grated.

Bowtie Pasta with Turkey Sausage

I've had it for dinner alone with out anything on the side and it was great. Some say you can serve it cold as a lunch or even as a salad but I have not tried it that way. (*I just love it as a dinner*) I also like to mix the pastas instead of just one. Use that corkscrew looking pasta or the one that looks like a butterfly.

Prep Time: 20 minutes
Cook Time: 20 minutes
Servings: 4

1 pound spicy turkey sausage, casings removed so we can separate it.
1 pound Farfalle pasta, whole wheat or Barilla Plus (multigrain)
1 cup mushrooms, sliced
1 cup canned cannellini beans, drained and rinsed
1 large bunch escarole(or Bok Choy), chopped course, (5 cups)
3 cloves garlic chopped fine
¼ cup chicken broth
⅛ teaspoon red pepper flakes
½ teaspoon ground pepper
½ teaspoon salt
¼ cup parmesan cheese, grated
¼ cup parsley leaves

In a large skillet heat olive oil over high heat. Add the mushrooms and cook till golden, about 3 minutes, set aside. Add sausage to same pan, breaking apart with a wooden spoon. Cook until brown, about 8 minutes. Return mushrooms to pan, add pepper flakes, add beans and stir. Add escarole, garlic, chicken broth, cover, turn heat to low and simmer about 7 or 8 more minutes until escarole wilts.

In large sauce pan boil water with a little salt, once boiling add pasta until tender but firm, about 8 minutes. Drain but keep 1 cup of the water in which you boiled the pasta.

In a large bowl put the pasta, add sausage mixture, salt, pepper and stir. Add a little of the pasta water, just ¼ cup to moisten. If you need more water add. Add parmesan cheese, toss, serve in small bowls, garnish with parsley leaves.

Side Dishes, Sauces

Side dishes to go with your dinner can be varied. Personally I like to just saute vegetables and maybe a sweet potato or some brown or wild rice. *(There is a lot of great rices in boxes now.)*

You can always steam some asparagus, broccoli or cauliflower in a small saucepan with just a ½ of an inch of water. Add salt, pepper and smart balance to taste and serve.

How about on the barbecue grill? Grill either asparagus, peppers, eggplant, onions, mushrooms, zucchini or yellow squash. Just brush a little olive oil on top. Use a screen over the grill to avoid losing those veggies to the coals. Yummy !

Many times I will toss a salad to eat before dinner and just have the main course by itself without a side dish.

From the following you can decide which side dish to have with each dinner. I think all of them work well together.

Sauteed Shiitake Mushrooms

Prep Time : 5 minutes
Cook time: 5 minutes
Servings: 2

2 tablespoons olive oil
¾ cup sliced shiitake mushrooms
1 tablespoon sesame oil
2 tablespoons lite soy sauce
2 tablespoon sake
1 orange, zested and juiced

Place a saute pan over medium-high heat. Add the oil and heat. When the oil is hot, add the mushrooms and saute until they begin to give up their liquid, about 4 minutes. Add the sesame oil, soy sauce, sake, orange juice and zest and cook for 2 additional minutes.

Serving with a slice of orange on the side.

Barbecue Sauces

These are low in fat and first rate in taste. They can be used with beef, pork or chicken. Pick the flavor you like. Each makes about 2 to 3 cups so you will have plenty for your meal and some leftover for the frig.

Prep Time: 10 minutes
Cook Time; 15 minutes

Traditional:
2 teaspoons canola or olive oil
¼ cup onion, chopped
2 cups ketchup
⅓ cup brown sugar substitute (Sugar Twin)
3 tablespoons worcestershire sauce
2 tablespoons lemon juice
Tabasco hot sauce to taste or any other hot sauce you may love.

Heat oil in a medium saucepan over high heat, add onion and /or garlic, cook 2 minutes. Stir in the remaining ingredients, bring to boil, reduce heat to low and simmer, covered, for 10 minutes.

Mexican:
2 teaspoons canola or olive oil
1 clove garlic, chopped fine or pressed
2 cups ketchup
⅓ cup brown sugar substitute (Sugar Twin)
3 tablespoons worcestershire sauce
¼ cup lime juice
1 can, small (4 oz) chopped green chilies, drained
2 tablespoons chili powder
1 ½ teaspoons ground cumin

Heat oil in a medium saucepan over high heat, add onion and /or garlic, cook 2 minutes. Stir in the remaining ingredients, bring to boil, reduce heat to low and simmer, covered, for 10 minutes.

Sweet, Smoky:
2 teaspoons canola or olive oil
¼ cup onion chopped
1 ½ cup ketchup
3 tablespoons worcestershire sauce
2 tablespoon cider vinegar
½ cup honey
1 teaspoon prepared mustard
½ teaspoon cayenne pepper
Hot sauce to taste

Heat oil in a medium saucepan over high heat, add onion and /or garlic, cook 2 minutes. Stir in the remaining ingredients, bring to boil, reduce heat to low and simmer, covered, for 10 minutes.

Fresh Spinach with Pine Nuts & Apricots

Yea, Yea, I know what your saying " NO, no, not spinach" but this one is good *(Bet you've heard that one before?)* This recipe came from Anne Stevenson. I was at her house visiting and saw her making it on the stove in about 5 minutes. When I tasted it I was impressed. Try it !

Prep Time: 5 minutes
Cook Time: 6 minutes

1 package fresh spinach, (12 ounce size)
⅓ cup pine nuts, toasted
½ cup dried apricots, chopped into pieces about ¼ inch square
2 tablespoons olive oil
1 clove garlic, chopped
3 tablespoon Balsamic vinegar
Salt and Pepper to taste

In a medium saucepan heat the oil and saute the garlic for about 2 to 3 minutes, add the spinach, stir, add Balsamic Vinegar. Turn heat down to medium and let the spinach reduce then add pine nuts and apricots. Sprinkle with salt and pepper.

Serve next to a chicken breast, steak or what have you. Good with everything.

Flowered Onions

There a little unusual but perfect as a side dish for your grilled steak or chicken.

Prep Time: 10 minutes
Cook Time: 25 to 30 minutes

4 medium to large sweet yellow onions
¼ cup Balsamic vinegar
⅛ cup olive oil
1 cup water
⅓ cup croutons, chopped or a slice of whole wheat bread, toasted and chopped small.
Parmesan cheese grated to taste.

Take the onions and cut ½ inch off the top and just a little off the bottom so it will sit without falling over. Then cut each onion into wedges (6 or 8) to within ½ inch from the bottom.
Put the onions in a microwavable dish with the water and micro on high 6 minutes.

Place each onion in the center of a piece of aluminum foil (about 12" long) brushed with a bit of olive oil where the onion sits. Wrap the foil up a bit around the onion. Then brush the onions with the mixture of balsamic vinegar and olive oil. Shape the foil completely around the onion now and twist to seal the top.

Place on barbecue grill for 15 or 20 minutes. I like putting the onions and juice in a individual bowl for each person sprinkled with the croutons and maybe some parmesan cheese.

Grilled Vegetables in Foil

This is one of my ultimate favorite vegetable dishes. I originally got it from a friend of mine in Kentucky. I do it all by memory so this is the first time it has been written down. Sorry Larry if I don't get it right. *(I am sure Larry will chastise me if I get it wrong)*

Prep Time: 20 minutes
Cook Time: About an hour on the bar-b

This is one of those, "what do you have in the refrigerator" recipes. If you don't have the following vegetables then substitute.

1 green pepper, sliced ¼ to ½ inch, seeds removed
1 large onion, sliced then slices cut in half
½ yellow squash
½ zucchini
½ head cabbage sliced
2 plum tomatoes or 6 or 7 cherry tomatoes
¾ cup broccoli flowerets
¾ cup mushrooms
2 or 3 tablespoons worcestershire sauce
3 tablespoons smart balance
¼ cup white wine.
Salt and pepper to taste

Lay out a 2 foot long piece of heavy duty tinfoil, then double it. Lay all the vegetables on the tin foil and turn up the sides. Place the rest of the ingredients on top of the vegetables. Now bring the sides up on the foil and make a sealed tent. Be sure there are no leaks.

Lay on barbecue grill on low heat to one side for 50 minutes to 1 hour. Be careful when opening as steam can burn. Serve on a platter and let people dish out from the tin foil.

Eggplant with Cinnamon and Cumin

This side dish goes great with just some plain grilled chicken breasts or even a nice grilled steak.

Prep Time: 10 minutes
Cook Time: 10 minutes
4 small Eggplants sliced ¼ inch thick
4 tablespoons olive oil
3 cloves garlic, chopped fine
2 onions diced
5 plum tomatoes, peeled, and diced
2 tablespoons honey
2 tablespoons cumin
1 tablespoon turmeric
1 tablespoon paprika
1 cinnamon stick
1 tablespoon red wine vinegar
2 tablespoons fresh cilantro, chopped
1 tablespoon fresh parsley, chopped
Salt to taste

Place the eggplant in a colander and toss with a little salt and let drain. Heat 2 tablespoons oil and brown eggplant in a skillet under high heat. Put aside.

In the same pan heat 2 more tablespoons oil and saute garlic, onions until translucent, add tomatoes, honey, spices (including cinnamon stick) and then eggplant. Cook until liquid is evaporated. Remove cinnamon stick and ad vinegar. Toss with cilantro and parsley and serve.

Brown Rice with Mushrooms

Prep Time: 15 min
Cook Time: 50 min
Servings: 6

2 tablespoon smart balance
¼ cup onion, chopped
1 garlic clove, minced
1 cup sliced mushrooms
¼ cup white wine
¾ teaspoon thyme
1 bay leaf
1 cup brown rice
2 cups chicken broth

In 3 quart sauce pan saute onion and garlic in the smart balance till the onions are translucent. (about 3 minutes) Add mushrooms, season with salt & pepper. Stir till mushrooms release their liquid, (about 2 to 3 min) Add wine stirring into mushrooms. Season with thyme and add bay leaf. Stir in rice until wine is absorbed then add ½ cup of chicken broth, turn heat down to low simmer leaving rice uncovered. Add more chicken broth as rice absorbs. Continue cooking until all the broth is gone and rice is cooked 'al dente'. Approximately 40 minutes.

Tomato Shells with Orzo & Parmesan

One of my wife's recipes that she has been making for years. A great side dish for any meat.

Prep Time: 15 min
Cook Time: 25 min

4 large tomatoes
1 cup dried orzo pasta
3 cups chicken broth
2 Tablespoons olive oil
½ cup onion, chopped
1 garlic clove, chopped
2 Tablespoons fresh basil minced or 1 teaspoon dried basil
½ cup grated parmesan cheese
salt and pepper to taste

Slice the tops off the tomatoes and keep on side. Scoop out the meat of the tomatoes chop well and place in medium size bowl. Sprinkle inside of tomatoes with salt & pepper and a pinch of basil.

In a sauce pan bring the 3 cups of chicken broth to a boil and add the orzo to cook. About 6 to 8 minutes. Drain orzo and reserve on side.

In a medium sauce pan saute onions and garlic in olive oil till onions are translucent (about 3 minutes) add reserved chopped tomatoes ½ the rest of basil. Add cooked drained orzo stirring well. Sprinkle in all but 2 tablespoons of parmesan cheese and blend together. Remove from heat.

Preheat oven to 350 degrees F. Place tomatoes in oven safe dish or pan. Fill tomatoes with orzo mixture, sprinkle the reserved parmesan on top. Place the tops of tomatoes on each and bake till heated through. (about 20 minutes. Serve warm.

If you want, make this as a complete meal. When you saute the onions and garlic add low fat chopped beef and cook before adding the rest of the mixture.

Asian Slaw

This is a great side dish for dinners like whole snapper, or baked flounder or even a crabmeat crepe.

Prep Time: 10 minutes
Serves: 4

½ cup each of the vegetables below. Julienne.
Carrots
Zucchini
Yellow Squash
Red Bell Pepper
Celery
Red Cabbage

Combine the above with the poppy seed dressing below.

¼ cup Rice Wine Vinegar
¼ cup cider Vinegar
2 packages Sweet & Low or Equal
1 tablespoon Sesame oil
1 tablespoon Olive oil
1 tablespoon poppy seeds

Combine all except oils and mix with wire whisk. Add oils and whisk well before combining with julienne vegetables.

Butternut Squash, Sweet & Sour

Prep Time: 30 minutes
Cook Time: 20 minutes
Servings: 4 to 6

2 butternut squash, cut into 1-inch slices, skin on, seeds discarded
4 tablespoons extra-virgin olive oil
¼ cup red wine vinegar
½ medium red onion, sliced paper-thin
½ teaspoon red chili flakes
1 tablespoons dried oregano
1 clove garlic, sliced paper-thin
Salt and pepper, to taste
¼ cup fresh mint leaves

Preheat oven to 450 degrees F. Place the sliced squash on a cookie sheet layered with tin foil. Season with a little salt and pepper to taste. Drizzle on 2 tablespoons of olive oil. Bake for 20 minutes or till tender.

In small bowl stir the remaining two tablespoons olive oil, vinegar, onion, chili flakes, oregano and garlic and season with more salt and pepper.

Remove squash from the oven and pour marinade over.

Allow to cool 20 minutes in the marinade, sprinkle with mint leaves and serve.

Stuffed Peppers with Olives

Prep Time: 15 minutes
Cook time: 30 minutes
Servings: 4

4 large yellow or red bell peppers and seeded yet left intact
½ cup golden raisins
toast 4 slices whole wheat bread in the toaster and crumble.
½ cup capers, rinsed
4 ounces green olives, pitted and coarsely chopped
4 cloves garlic, crushed and minced
1 cup grated parmesan or pecorino
2 tablespoons extra-virgin olive oil
Salt and pepper, to taste
1 cup red wine
2 tablespoons sherry vinegar

In a large bowl, combine the raisins, crumbled bread, capers, olives, garlic, cheese, oil, salt and pepper and mix well with hands to form a smooth mixture. Divide the mixture into 4 equal portions and stuff each pepper. Be sure not to tear the sides of the peppers.

Preheat your oven to 375 degrees F. In a shallow casserole place the peppers and pour the wine and the vinegar around the stuffed peppers. Cook in the oven for 30 minutes, until just starting to darken, basting occasionally with the wine/ sherry vinegar mixture.

Serve immediately, or cool and serve at room temperature, your choice. They're good both ways.

Snacks, Finger Food, Party Food

Just because you're going through a lifestyle change in the way you eat, it does not mean you can't party and have a good time. My wife has been making low fat, low sugar party snacks for years. I can tell you that everyone, and I mean everyone, loves her parties. (*maybe the booze has a little to do with it*)

The way to stay with this lifestyle is to be happy with it. I feel if I can give you delicious food to eat at any time you will stick with it.

Sometimes in the middle of the day when those cravings start or you just want to have something to eat. I feel the same way and usually have a bowl of fruit but having one of the following snacks is not going to hurt you. Make them up in advance and put them in the refrigerator. For the ones that have to be warmed the microwave does a pretty good job. I personally do not like the micro for cooking but heating is OK.

For a snack, if you can just have a bite or two, try one of the low fat, sugar free snack bars I mentioned under 'Let's go Shopping'.

Asian Snapper Bites

Easy finger food is necessary when having friends over and this recipe fits the bill. Leave the fish to marinate while you prepare the rest of the food and simply grill before guests arrive.

Prep Time: 30 minutes
Cooking Time: 10 minutes
Ready in: 40 minutes
Servings: 20 pieces

2 tbsp soy sauce, reduced salt
2 tbsp lime juice
1 knob ginger peeled and shredded
½ tsp sesame oil
1 kg (2 pounds) red snapper cut into cubes approx. 1 inch thick

Combine the soy, lime juice and ginger together. Pour over the fish and leave to marinate for 30 minutes.
Thread 2 pieces of the fish on small soaked bamboo skewers and grill for 6 - 8 minutes or saute in a pan heated with the sesame oil, turning once.

Tastes great with many dipping sauces.

Shrimp Sates with Spiced Chutney

Prep Time: 40 minutes
Cook Time: 1 hour 30 minutes
Servings: About 32 hor d'oeuvres

1 1/4 pounds deveined shelled shrimp (about 32)
1 tablespoon minced garlic
3 tablespoons olive oil
2 tablespoons fresh lime juice

Butterfly shrimp by cutting almost, but not all the way, through backs. Toss with garlic, oil, and lime juice. Season with salt. Marinate, chilled, 1 hour.
Preheat broiler
Gently press 1 shrimp open and thread lengthwise onto a bamboo skewer near pointed end. Repeat with remaining shrimp and skewers.

Arrange satis in a row on 1 long side of a broiler pan so that blunt ends of skewers point toward middle of pan. Cover exposed portions of skewers with a sheet of foil (don't cover shrimp). Arrange another row of satis over foil. Continue adding rows of satis and layers of foil until pan is full, making sure exposed skewer ends of last row of satis are covered with foil.
Broil until shrimp are just cooked through, 3 to 4 minutes. Serve satis with chutney for dipping.
CHUTNEY:
1 (16-ounce) container plain fat free yogurt
2 teaspoons ground coriander
1 teaspoon ground cumin
1 tablespoon olive oil
4 fresh jalapeno chile's, 3 with seeds and ribs removed
2 cups fresh cilantro sprigs
2 tablespoons fresh lime juice

To make chutney: Drain yogurt in a fine-mesh sieve set over a bowl, chill, 1 hour. Cook coriander and cumin in oil in a small skillet over moderate heat, stirring occasionally, until fragrant. Coarsely chop chile's, then puree in a blender with drained yogurt, coriander mixture, and cilantro until smooth. Stir in lime juice and salt to taste.

147

SUPER HOT - HOT WINGS (MARDY'S FAMOUS)

The following recipe is from my wife. They are so good it's almost criminal

Prep time: 20 minutes
Cooking time: 35 minutes
Servings: 2 real hungry people or 4 normal people

8	chicken wings, wing tip removed
4	tablespoons smart balance
4	tablespoons tabasco
1	tablespoon ketchup
1	garlic clove minced
½	teaspoon cumin

Cut the eight wings in half making 16 pieces

Place in non stick small roasting pan and bake in preheated 400 degree oven for 40 minutes turning once.

Place smart balance in sauce pan and melt, add garlic, stir, add tabasco, ketchup and cumin. Stir until blended and remove from heat.

When the wings are cooked remove from oven and pour sauce over stirring to coat. Place back into oven for 5 minutes.

Serve on some lettuce leaves with low fat ranch dressing on side. Personally, I just like them the way they are.

If you find the sauce too hot for your taste lessen the tabasco sauce.

Tortilla Swirls

Prep Time: 15 minutes
Cooking Time: none
Servings: 12

9 Fat Free flour Tortillas (6 inch)
¾ cup nonfat cream cheese
½ cup nonfat sour cream
1 cup shredded nonfat cheddar or jack cheese
½ green pepper chopped fine
8 scallions, thin sliced
2 teaspoons lime juice
¼ cup salsa

In a small bowl beat cream cheese, sour cream until smooth with electric mixer. Blend in cheddar (or jack) cheese, pepper, scallions and lime juice.

Spread about ¼ cup of the cheese mixture on each tortilla, roll up with plastic wrap and refrigerate until chilled.

With serrated knife, cut each roll into 6 equal slices. Arrange on serving platter, top each swirl with ¼ teaspoon salsa.

Note: In addition or for a change add spinach to the tortillas prior to rolling and cutting. Also, low fat sliced lunchmeats, turkey or chicken, add a great protein boost.

Mushrooms stuffed with Spinach

Prep Time: 15 minutes
Cook time: 30 minutes
Servings: 24 mushrooms, serves 8 people

24 large white mushrooms
¼ cup chopped shallots or onions
2 cloves garlic, chopped fine
2 tablespoons balsamic vinegar
1 tablespoon Italian seasoning
¼ cup water
10 ounces chopped fresh spinach

Wash mushrooms, remove stems. Lay out caps in non stick pan and put in 350 degree oven for 5 to 10 minutes to cook slightly. Set aside.

Chop mushroom stems fine.

Saute shallots (onions), garlic and balsamic vinegar in small saucepan. When onions are translucent add chopped mushroom stems, water and seasoning. Cook 2 to 3 minutes. Add spinach and cook till water is almost evaporated.

Mound the mixture in the mushroom caps. Bake for 10 to 15 minutes until hot.

Cucumber Salsa

Prep Time: 10 minutes
Serves: 4

1 cup diced cucumber
½ cup orange sections, chopped
¼ cup red onion, chopped
1 tablespoon fresh orange juice
2 tablespoons jalapeno peppers, chopped fine
1 tablespoon white wine vinegar
2 tablespoon olive oil
¼ teaspoon salt
⅛ teaspoon pepper

In a bowl combine all ingredients, stir well.

Serve chilled or at room temperature

Nutty Chicken Puffs

Great for a party. This recipe will make about 70. Good for you and great tasting.

Prep Time: 15 minutes
Cooking Time: 20 minutes
Servings: 10 to 12

1 ½ cups skinless boneless chicken breast, chopped fine
½ cup almonds, chopped and toasted
1 cup chicken broth
⅓ cup olive oil
2 teaspoons worcestershire sauce
1 tablespoon parsley, chopped fine
½ teaspoon seasoned salt
1 teaspoon celery seed
⅛ teaspoon cayenne pepper
½ cup whole wheat flour
½ cup all purpose flour
1 cup egg substitute

In a bowl combine the chicken and almonds, set aside

In a large saucepan combine the chicken broth, almonds, olive oil, worcestershire sauce, parsley, salt and celery seed. Bring to a boil, Add flour all at once, stir until a smooth ball forms, remove and let stand for 5 minutes.

In a large bowl place the saucepan mixture add egg substitute beating well until smooth, stir in chicken and almonds.

Preheat oven to 450 degrees. On a greased baking sheet drop heaping teaspoons. Bake for 13 to 15 minutes until brown.

Serve warm.

Taco Dip

This is a nice creamy dip. Be sure to use the low fat baked tortilla chips when you serve.

Prep Time: 15 minutes
Servings: 8

2 -8 ounce packages or fat free cream cheese
1 teaspoon taco seasoning
1 teaspoon parsley chopped
1 cup chunky salsa (look for the low sugar, low fat variety)
⅓ cup shredded reduced fat cheddar cheese
⅓ cup pitted olives chopped. (green or black to your taste)

In a medium bowl stir cream cheese with a spoon until soft, stir in taco seasoning, parsley and salsa, mix. Add cheddar cheese and olives, mix well.

Cover and refrigerate for about an hour.

Serve with the tortilla chips.

Chickpea and Roasted Red Pepper Dip

You can serve this with fresh vegetables like broccoli, sliced yellow squash, baby carrots and cauliflower or with baked tortilla chips.

Prep Time: 10 minutes
Servings: 16

16 ounces canned chickpeas, rinsed and drained
7 ounces roasted red pepper, rinsed and drained
½ cup nonfat yogurt, no flavoring
2 cloves garlic, chopped
¼ teaspoon salt
¼ teaspoon pepper

Process all of the above in a food processor or blender until smooth. Serve in bowl.

Egg Rolls

Prep Time: 15 minutes
Cook Time: 30 minutes
Serves: 8

8 egg roll wrappers
1 head chinese cabbage, shredded, outer leaves removed.
2 carrots shredded
2 garlic cloves, minced
2 scallions, chopped. Use all of the scallion, white and green
1 tablespoon ginger, fresh, minced.
1 tablespoon low sodium soy sauce
2 teaspoons cornstarch
1 teaspoon sesame oil
A little olive oil to coat egg rolls with brush or olive oil cooking spray

Place cabbage in a microwavable dish and cover. Microwave on high until wilted, about 4 minutes, drain and transfer to a large bowl.

Add the carrots, garlic, scallions, ginger, soy sauce, cornstarch and sesame oil, mix well.

Preheat oven to 350 degrees.

Lay out egg roll wrappers on a clean, dry surface. Spoon cabbage mixture diagonally onto each wrapper. Fold over one of the corners to cover the filling. Fold up the other two corners. Moisten edge of remaining corner with water and roll up wrapper like a jellyroll.

Brush egg rolls with just a little olive oil.

Spray a baking sheet with cooking spray or brush with olive oil. Place egg rolls on and bake for 25 minutes.

Serve hot.

Soups

Oriental Hot 'n' Sour Soup

Prep Time: 10 Minutes
Cook Time: 30 Minutes
Ready In: 40 Minutes
Servings: 4

INGREDIENTS:
4 cups chicken broth
2-1/2 slices fresh ginger root
1/2 teaspoon whole black peppercorns
3 fresh green onions, chopped
1/2 red bell pepper, diced
1/2 cup fresh sliced mushrooms
1/4 cup bamboo shoots
1/4 cup rice vinegar
1 teaspoon chili powder
1 teaspoon sesame oil

DIRECTIONS:
In a large cooking pot, add chicken broth, ginger root, and peppercorns, and bring to boil. Reduce heat to low and simmer uncovered for 20 minutes.
Strain broth, discard ginger root and peppercorns. Return strained broth to pot. Add green onions, red pepper, mushrooms, bamboo shoots, rice wine vinegar, chili powder, and sesame oil. Simmer for 10 minutes or until vegetables are just tender.

Fresh Mushroom Soup

Prep Time: 10 minutes
Cook time: 20 minutes
Servings: 4

¾ to 1 pound wild mushrooms sliced.
2 onions, chopped
2 tablespoons smart balance
½ cup water
6 cups beef broth
½ to ¾ cups fat free sour cream
3 tablespoons flour
½ teaspoon black pepper
3 tablespoons chopped parsley.

In a soup pot or large saucepan saute mushrooms and onions in smart balance and a little water until they're cooked through, add 5 cups beef broth.

In a separate bowl, blend sour cream and flour with 1 cup of broth until lump free. Add to soup slowly, simmer 10 minutes add pepper.

Serve in soup bowls and garnish with parsley.

Coconut Chicken Soup (Thai)

Prep Time:15 Minutes
Cook Time:20 Minutes
Ready In:35 Minutes
Servings:6

INGREDIENTS:
3/4 pound boneless, skinless chicken meat
3 tablespoons vegetable oil
2 (14 ounce) cans coconut milk
2 cups water
2 tablespoons minced fresh ginger root
4 tablespoons fish sauce (available in ethnic food isle of your store)
1/4 cup fresh lime juice
1/4 tablespoon cayenne pepper
1/2 teaspoon ground turmeric
2 tablespoons thinly sliced green onion
1 tablespoon chopped fresh cilantro

DIRECTIONS:
Cut chicken into thin strips and saute in oil for to 2 to 3 minutes until the chicken turns white.

In a pot, bring coconut milk and water to a boil. Reduce heat. Add ginger, fish sauce, lime juice, cayenne pepper and turmeric. Simmer until the chicken is done, 10 to 15 minutes.

Sprinkle with scallions and fresh cilantro and serve steaming hot.

TOMATO SOUP WITH GOAT'S CHEESE DUMPLINGS
(Dumplings on next page)

I feel this soup is a complete meal with the dumplings. Please don't have this the first month on our program. Wait till you have stabilized your insulin and digestive system.

Prep Time: 30 minutes
Cooking Time: 1 hour 30 minutes
Servings: 6 to 8

2 tablespoons olive oil
2 cups chopped yellow onions
1 cup chopped celery
1 cup chopped carrots
2 tablespoons minced garlic
8 cups chopped fresh tomatoes, peeled and seeded
8 cups chicken broth
¼ cup finely chopped parsley
Salt and pepper
Pinch of cayenne

In a large sauce pan, heat the olive oil. When the oil is hot, saute the onions, celery and carrots. Season with salt, pepper, and cayenne. Saute for 4 to 5 minutes. Add the garlic and tomatoes. Cook for 3 to 4 minutes, stirring often. Add the chicken broth and bring to a boil. Reduce the heat to a simmer and cook for 1 hour and 15 minutes.

Using a hand-held blender, puree the soup in the pan. Stir in ½ the parsley. Add a little salt and pepper if needed.

GOAT CHEESE DUMPLINGS

You can use these dumplings in other soups also. You can even bake them on a cookie sheet for appetizers.

1 cup Goat's cheese (cheve), room temperature
2 tablespoons extra-virgin olive oil
2 tablespoons finely chopped basil
16 wonton wrappers found in the fresh produce area of your store
1/4 cup water

In a small mixing bowl, combine the Goat's cheese, extra-virgin olive oil and basil. Mix until the mixture is smooth. Season with salt and pepper.

Spoon 1 tablespoon of the cheese mixture in the center of each wonton wrapper. Brush the edges of the wrappers with a little water. Bring two corners of the wrappers together and seal, forming a triangle.

In a small sauce pan with boiling water poach the dumplings for 2 to 3 minutes or until the dumplings float. Remove and drain on a paper-lined plate.

Season the dumplings with some pepper. In a shallow bowl place two dumplings and ladle in the soup mixture.

Garnish with the rest of the parsley.

A Good Peasant Soup

A soup that really makes a good lunch or a pre dinner soup if your having a large family meal. Serve with a hearty whole grain bread.

Prep Time: 15 minutes
Cook Time: 10 minutes
Servings: 4 to 6

2 carrots sliced in ¼ inch rounds
⅔ cup onion chopped
½ pound cooked turkey sausage (smoked turkey or kielbasa turkey links) sliced in ¼ inch slices then halved
2 cloves garlic sliced thin or chopped fine
3 cans chicken broth (I like the low sodium kind)
2 cans cannellini beans drained and rinsed
4 cups fresh baby spinach
1 tablespoon olive oil
black pepper to taste

In a 4 quart saucepan heat oil till hot, add garlic, onion, sausage, carrots, stir for 5 or 6 minutes until vegetables are cooked crisp. Add chicken broth, cover and bring to boil.

Remove from heat stir in the beans and spinach, cover and let stand 3 to 5 minutes before serving.

Onion Soup from Central Italy

Prep Time: 30 minutes
Cook Time: 35 minutes
Servings: 4

¼ cup diced pancetta ham or low fat baked ham
1 tablespoon Olive oil
4 onions thinly sliced into rings
3 Garlic cloves chopped
3 ½ cup chicken broth
4 slices sourdough bread
2 tablespoons Smart Balance
3 ounces low fat swiss cheese in slices
Salt and pepper

Dry fry the pancetta (or ham) in a large saucepan for 3-4 minutes until it begins to brown. Remove from the pan and set aside until required.

Add the oil to the pan and cook the onions and garlic over a high heat for 4 minutes. Reduce the heat, cover, and cook for 15 minutes, or until the onions are lightly caramelized.

Add the chicken broth to the saucepan and bring to a boil. Reduce the heat and leave mixture to simmer, covered, for about 10 minutes.

Toast the slices of sourdough bread until golden. Spread the sourdough bread with the Smart Balance and top with the swiss cheese. Place in broiler and heat till cheese melts. Remove and cut the bread into bite-size pieces. Add the reserved pancetta (or ham) to the soup and season with salt and pepper to taste.

Pour into soup bowls and top with the toasted bread and melted cheese.

Sweet Potato Soup

Prep Time: 15 minutes
Cook Time: 40 minutes
Servings: 6 to 8

1 onion, chopped
2 stalks celery, chopped
3 pounds sweet potatoes, peeled and diced
8 cups chicken broth
1 tablespoon curry powder (use mild if you like, I prefer hot)
2 teaspoons thyme
1 teaspoon freshly ground black or white pepper
⅛ teaspoon cayenne, to taste
¼ cup brandy (optional) (*not optional for me, that's the good part*)
2 cups soy milk

Combine the onion, celery, sweet potatoes, chicken broth, curry powder and thyme in a large pot. Bring to a boil, reduce the heat and simmer, 30-40 minutes, or until the potatoes are soft.

With a slotted spoon, remove about 2 cups of the vegetables and set aside. Puree the remaining soup with a hand blender until it is fairly smooth.

Return the vegetables to the pot, stir in the brandy and soy milk, and heat through.

Serve

Wild Mushroom Soup

This is a tasty soup with a real mushroom taste. It makes enough for two meals so you can freeze some for later if you wish.

Prep Time: 20 minutes
Cook Time: 40 minutes
Serves: 12

3 quarts chicken broth
½ lb. portobello mushrooms cut into small cubes
¼ lb. shiitake mushrooms thinly sliced
¼ lb. oyster mushrooms thinly sliced
If you cant find the above mushrooms, substitute with what you have.
1 oz. low-sodium soy sauce
½ teaspoon curry powder
3 cloves garlic minced
½ teaspoon white pepper
¼ cup Smart Balance
¼ teaspoon dried basil leaves
½ teaspoon seasoned salt
1 shot of scotch whiskey, bourbon is good also
¼ teaspoon black pepper
⅛ teaspoon cayenne pepper
6 oz. angel hair pasta

In stockpot, bring chicken broth to boil. Add portobello mushrooms, shiitake and oyster mushrooms. Add soy sauce, curry powder, garlic powder, white pepper, Smart Balance, basil, salt, scotch, freshly ground pepper and cayenne. Continue boiling for 10 minutes.

Reduce heat and simmer for 25 minutes. Add angel hair and cook briefly until pasta is cooked through, about 4 to 5 minutes.

Serve

Zucchini and Cheese Soup

Prep time: 15 minutes
Cook Time: 15 minutes
Servings: 4

2 cups finely chopped onion
3 Tablespoons Smart Balance
6 regular or 12 small zucchini cut julienne
1 teaspoon dried rosemary crushed
4 cups chicken broth
½ teaspoon salt
½ teaspoon pepper
1 teaspoon Splenda
1 cup fat free light cream or half and half
2 cups grated low fat cheddar cheese, monterey jack works also
fresh chives chopped for garnish

Saute the onions in Smart Balance until translucent in large saucepan.
Add the zucchini and rosemary. Do not let zucchini get completely soft.

Place ½ the mixture in blender and puree. Add puree back to pan with
the chicken stock, cheese, salt and sugar. Bring to a slight boil stirring for
5 minutes. Reduce heat and add cream/ or half and half stirring through
out so cream soup mixture does not boil. Continue until warmed
through.

Serve with chives on top.

Dessert (YES!)

Desserts are not on the top of our list of foods for you to eat. I know, I know, I like the desserts myself. What I do is buy Sugar Free Jello. Lime, strawberry, mixed berry, whatever you can find. If you don't like the jello straight out of the box then mix in some fresh fruit.

I also enjoy sugar free instant pudding. My favorite is to mix up a box of Pistachio and a box of Chocolate. Then pour ½ a small serving bowl with chocolate and top it with the pistachio, Yum.

Another great dessert straight from the old country, Cheese! Europe where many finish their meals with a plate of assorted cheeses and fruit. My suggestion is to cut up some low fat cheese and an apple. You won't believe how good an apple goes with cheddar, swiss or monterey jack. Another trick is to eat grapes with the cheese.

Another European favorite is to have your salad after your meal. I have tried it many times and really like it. It fills you up quite nicely.

Sugar free Ice Cream seems to be ok with some people, others do not lose weight eating it. This may be due to the amount consumed. (*I know that's my problem*) Do not have this in the first month, but after you can try a scoop or two and see if you keep losing at the same rate.

Try fresh raspberries or strawberries with a little fat free, sugar free topping like Cool Whip.

Nuts are good for you also if you don't overdo it. Have 10 or 12 almonds or 15 or 20 peanuts for dessert.

The following desserts are for your enjoyment but remember, like anything, don't overdue it.

Ricotta Cheese with Almonds & Walnuts

Prep Time: 10 minutes
Serves: 2

1 cup part skim ricotta cheese
2 packages sugar substitute
1 tablespoon slivered almonds, toasted
1 tablespoon walnuts chopped
½ teaspoon almond extract.

Mix the cheese, sugar substitute and extract in a bowl.

Chill in refrigerator and serve with slivered almonds and walnuts sprinkled on top.

Ricotta Cheese and Orange

Same as the above recipe except substitute vanilla extract for the almond extract and substitute orange zest for the slivered almonds. I like squeezing just a little fresh orange juice in also.

Pears with Ginger

Prep Time: 10 minutes
Cooking Time: 25 minutes
Servings: 4 to 6

4 medium size pears, cored, peeled and cut in half
½ cup crushed gingersnaps
¼ cup fresh 100% orange juice
2 tablespoons walnuts, chopped
2 tablespoon almonds chopped
2 tablespoons smart balance

Place the pear halves, cut side up in a 11" x 9" oven proof baking dish. Pour orange juice over each pear.

In a bowl, combine gingersnaps, walnuts, smart balance and sprinkle over pears.

Bake in a 350 degree preheated oven for 25 minutes.

Strawberries with Balsamic

Prep Time: 10 minutes
Servings: 4

1 quart strawberries. Take the stem off and halve them.
4 tablespoons balsamic vinegar
2 packages sugar substitute like Equal or Sweet and Low
⅛ teaspoon Black Pepper
Mint leafs for garnish

In a bowl combine the strawberries, sugar substitute, balsamic vinegar. Let stand for a short while and toss again.

Serve in individual bowls, sprinkle pepper on top and garnish with mint.

Chewy Brownies

Prep time: 15 minutes
Cook time: 30 minutes
Servings: 16 brownies

2 oz. unsweetened chocolate at least 60% cocoa

¾ cup all-purpose flour

⅓ cup canola oil
½ tsp. baking powder

2 eggs

¼ tsp. salt

2 packages artificial sweetener or ¼ cup Splenda

½ cup coarsely chopped walnuts

1 tsp. vanilla extract

Heat oven to 325° F. Grease a 9-inch square baking pan; set aside.

Melt chocolate and oil in a medium saucepan over low heat. Remove from heat; beat in eggs, one at a time, until blended. Stir in sweetener and vanilla. Blend flour, baking powder, and salt; stir into chocolate mixture. Stir in nuts.

Spread mixture in greased pan. Bake 30 minutes. Cool in pan on a wire rack.

Cut into 16 bars.

Apple and Polenta Crumble

There's nothing more delicious than apple crumble. Not the same consistency as traditional crumble but better for you.

Preparation time: 20 minutes
Cooking time: 35 minutes
Servings: 6 (Well........... Maybe)

1 cup coarse polenta
2 cups water
1/4 cup apple concentrate
1/4 cup tahini sesame paste
1/4 cup olive oil
4 apples peeled and sliced, about a pound
1/2 teaspoon cinnamon
Vanilla low fat yogurt

Preheat the oven to 350°F. In a small pan combine the apple concentrate, tahini sesame paste, water and oil and slowly bring it to the boil stirring continuously. Add the polenta; reduce the heat to low and simmer, stirring constantly for 10 minutes. Set aside to cool.

Arrange the apples in the bottom of a pie dish and sprinkle with cinnamon. Using your hands, crumble the polenta over the top.

Bake for about 30 minutes.

For a really special dish serve with frozen yogurt on the side.

Baked Apple Sections with Orange

Prep Time: 10 minutes
Cook Time: 20 minutes

2 golden delicious apples cut into sections then halved. Use granny smith if you want the taste to be a bit tart.
10 or 12 grapes
1 small can of unsweetened pineapple chunks in juice
1 teaspoon smart balance
½ cup orange juice
1 orange sectioned
1 tablespoon orange zest
Cinnamon to taste.

In a ovenproof dish add smart balance, apples, pineapple, juice, grapes, oranges, zest and orange juice.

Sprinkle with cinnamon, cover and bake in a 350 degree oven for about 18 to 20 minutes.

Pears Stuffed with Chocolate

Prep time: 10 minutes
Cook Time: 20 minutes
Servings: 2

2 pears
16 semisweet chocolate chips
2 tablespoon slivered almonds

Slice the top off the pears just above the widest part. Scoop out the cores from the bottom halves with a small spoon. Fill the scooped out section with the semisweet chocolate chips. (8 in each) and some slivered almonds. Put the top back on the pear.

Stand each pear in a custard cup that is oven proof. Set the cups in a saucepan and add about an inch of water. Bring the water to point where it is just about to boil and turn down low. Cover, steam for about 20 min. Pears will turn translucent.

Serve warm.

Fresh Berry's with Yogurt and Chocolate

Prep & Cook Time: 10 minutes
Servings: 4

1 basket fresh raspberries or strawberries
8 ounces low fat vanilla yogurt
2 ounces melted dark chocolate (more than 60% cocoa)

Fold together yogurt and berries

Melt chocolate in a double boiler with heat on medium. Place berries and yogurt in individual bowls and drizzle with melted chocolate.

Baked Apple

This is easy and effortless to make. Serve it to company, they will love it.

Prep time: 10 minutes
Cook Time: 1 hour
Servings: 4

4 crisp red apples
2 tablespoons fresh lemon juice
2 cups water
½ cup sugar free maple syrup
½ cup raisins
½ cup walnuts
1 teaspoon cinnamon

Core apples using a melon baller leaving the bottom of apple so they hold the stuffing. Combine the lemon juice and water in a medium bowl and place apples in the mixture as you complete coring them.

In a small bowl mix the maple syrup, raisins, walnuts and cinnamon, mix. Fill apples with the mixture.

Place apples in a baking dish with about 1 cup of the lemon water. Bake uncovered for about an hour or until tender.

Put each apple in a small serving bowl and drizzle juice from the bottom of the pan over the apples and serve.

Blueberry and Peach Crisp

Easy to prepare and delicious. Serve this to anyone and they will love it. A little frozen yogurt on top for a variation.

Prep time: 10 minutes
Cook time: 45 minutes
Servings: 4

12 ounces fresh blueberries
1 pound fresh peach slices
¼ cup apple juice
2 tablespoons apple juice
½ cup almonds
½ cup oats
1 cup pitted dates
½ teaspoon cinnamon

Preheat oven to 350 degrees. Place blueberries in the bottom of a 8 inch baking dish. Place peach slices on top of the blueberries. Drizzle the ¼ cup apple juice over the top.

Remove pits from dates and place in a food processor along with the oats and cinnamon. Run for about a minute, add 2 tablespoons apple juice and mix.

Place mixture evenly over peaches and blueberries, bake uncovered for about 45 minutes.

Serve warm. I have also served it cold but I like it warm better.

Note: If the topping has a tendency to be in clumps after processing it then crumple it with your hands into an even layer.

Apricot Compote with Pears

You can serve it like the recipe states or with a little vanilla yogurt.

Prep time: 5 minutes
Cook Time: 10 minutes
Servings: 2

1 Pear sliced in half
1 cup dried apricots, sliced
½ cup raisins
½ cup chopped walnuts
2 tablespoons fresh lemon juice
1 ½ cups fresh orange juice
2 tablespoons honey

In a small saucepan bring the lemon juice, orange juice and honey to a boil, add apricots and raisins. Reduce heat to low and simmer until they become tender and a little syrupy. Usually about 10 minutes. Do not overcook.

Remove the apricots and raisins with a slotted spoon and let the mixture thicken for about 2 minutes.

Remove from heat and add the apricots, raisins, and walnuts into the sauce.

Place ½ pear in small serving bowl and spoon have the mixture over. Repeat with other pear half.

I like it served warm but you can serve it cold.

Blueberries, Yogurt and Peaches

A great summer recipe with fresh peaches and blueberries.

Prep Time: 10 minutes
Servings: 4

1 basket of fresh blueberries
4 fresh peaches sliced
4 ounces vanilla yogurt

In a small serving bowl lay out slices of peaches, place a little yogurt in the center and sprinkle blueberries on top.

This is not

The End

This is just the Beginning of your New Life

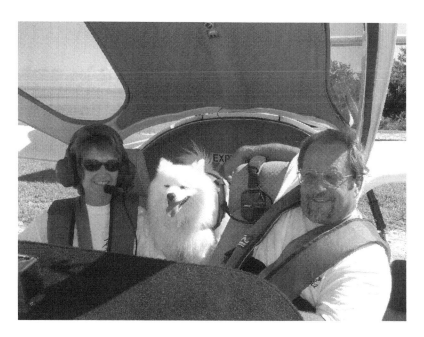

Wife Mardy, (super dog) Keiko, and author Paul Array
in their Experimental amphibious aircraft.

While competitive drag racing held Paul's attention for several award winning years, his love for the freedom of flight took him to even greater heights. An accomplished commercial pilot, with a degree in aeronautical engineering, Paul has thousands of hours as captain of both land and sea aircraft. Having retired from his private investigative agency, he turned to his second love, the sea, to fulfill his fondest dream, sailing to new and exciting places with his first love Mardy. Writing became a by product of his experience. Paul now lives in Key West, Florida with his wife Mardy and their furry child Keiko.

Notes

Notes

Notes

Made in the USA
Lexington, KY
06 July 2013